Thai in Vitro

Fertility, Reproduction and Sexuality

General Editors:

Soraya Tremayne, Founding Director, Fertility and Reproduction Studies Group, and Research Associate, Institute of Social and Cultural Anthropology, University of Oxford
Marcia C. Inhorn, William K. Lanman, Jr. Professor of Anthropology and International Affairs, Yale University
David Parkin, Fellow of All Souls College, University of Oxford
Philip Kreager, Director, Fertility and Reproduction Studies Group, and Research Associate, Institute of Social and Cultural Anthropology and Institute of Human Sciences, University of Oxford

Volume 1
Managing Reproductive Life: Cross-Cultural Themes in Fertility & Sexuality
Edited by Soraya Tremayne

Volume 2
Modern Babylon? Prostituting Children in Thailand
Heather Montgomery

Volume 3
Reproductive Agency, Medicine and the State: Cultural Transformations in Childbearing
Edited by Maya Unnithan-Kumar

Volume 4
A New Look at Thai AIDS: Perspectives from the Margin
Graham Fordham

Volume 5
Breast Feeding and Sexuality: Behaviour, Beliefs and Taboos among the Gogo Mothers in Tanzania
Mara Mabilia

Volume 6
Ageing without Children: European and Asian Perspectives on Elderly Access to Support Networks
Edited by Philip Kreager and Elisabeth Schröder-Butterfill

Volume 7
Nameless Relations: Anonymity, Melanesia and Reproductive Gift Exchange between British Ova Donors and Recipients
Monica Konrad

Volume 8
Population, Reproduction and Fertility in Melanesia
Edited by Stanley J. Ulijaszek

Volume 9
Conceiving Kinship: Assisted Conception, Procreation and Family in Southern Europe
Monica M. E. Bonaccorso

Volume 10
Where There is No Midwife: Birth and Loss in Rural India
Sarah Pinto

Volume 11
Reproductive Disruptions: Gender, Technology, and Biopolitics in the New Millennium
Edited by Marcia C. Inhorn

Volume 12
Reconceiving the Second Sex: Men, Masculinity, and Reproduction
Edited by Marcia C. Inhorn, Tine Tjørnhøj-Thomsen, Helene Goldberg and Maruska la Cour Mosegaard

Volume 13
Transgressive Sex: Subversion and Control in Erotic Encounters
Edited by Hastings Donnan and Fiona Magowan

Volume 14
European Kinship in the Age of Biotechnology
Edited by Jeanette Edwards and Carles Salazar

Volume 15
Kinship and Beyond: The Genealogical Model Reconsidered
Edited by Sandra Bamford and James Leach

Volume 16
Islam and New Kinship: Reproductive Technology and the Shariah in Lebanon
Morgan Clarke

Volume 17
Childbirth, Midwifery and Concepts of Time
Edited by Christine McCourt

Volume 18
Assisting Reproduction, Testing Genes: Global Encounters with the New Biotechnologies
Edited by Daphna Birenbaum-Carmeli and Marcia C. Inhorn

Volume 19
Kin, Gene, Community: Reproductive Technologies among Jewish Israelis
Edited by Daphna Birenbaum-Carmeli and Yoram S. Carmeli

Volume 20
Abortion in Asia: Local Dilemmas, Global Politics
Edited by Andrea Whittaker

Volume 21
Unsafe Motherhood: Mayan Maternal Mortality and Subjectivity in Post-War Guatemala
Nicole S. Berry

Volume 22
Fatness and the Maternal Body: Women's Experiences of Corporeality and the Shaping of Social Policy
Edited by Maya Unnithan-Kumar and Soraya Tremayne

Volume 23
Islam and Assisted Reproductive Technologies: Sunni and Shia Perspectives
Edited by Marcia C. Inhorn and Soraya Tremayne

Volume 24
Militant Lactivism? Attachment Parenting and Intensive Motherhood in the UK and France
Charlotte Faircloth

Volume 25
Pregnancy in Practice: Expectation and Experience in the Contemporary US
Sallie Han

Volume 26
Nighttime Breastfeeding: An American Cultural Dilemma
Cecília Tomori

Volume 27
Globalized Fatherhood
Edited by Marcia C. Inhorn, Wendy Chavkin, and José-Alberto Navarro

Volume 28
Cousin Marriages: Between Tradition, Genetic Risk and Cultural Change
Edited by Alison Shaw and Aviad Raz

Volume 29
Achieving Procreation: Childlessness and IVF in Turkey
Merve Demircioğlu Goknar

Volume 30
Thai in Vitro: Gender, Culture and Assisted Reproduction
Andrea Whittaker

THAI IN VITRO
Gender, Culture and Assisted Reproduction

Andrea Whittaker

berghahn
NEW YORK • OXFORD
www.berghahnbooks.com

First published in 2015 by

Berghahn Books

www.berghahnbooks.com

Library of Congress Cataloging-in-Publication Data

Whittaker, Andrea (Andrea M.), 1967– , author.
Thai in vitro : gender, culture and assisted reproduction / Andrea Whittaker.
p. ; cm. — (Fertility, reproduction and sexuality ; volume 30)
Includes bibliographical references and index.
ISBN 978-1-78238-732-9 (hardback : alk. paper) —
ISBN 978-1-78238-733-6 (ebook)
I. Title. II. Series: Fertility, reproduction, and sexuality ; v. 30.
[DNLM: 1. Fertilization in Vitro—trends—Thailand. 2. Culture—Thailand. 3. Infertility—psychology—Thailand. 4. Infertility—therapy—Thailand. 5. Socioeconomic Factors—Thailand. WQ 208]
RG135.W52 2015
362.1966'92009593—dc23

2014039963

British Library Cataloguing in Publication Data

A catalogue record for this book is available from the British Library.

Printed on acid-free paper

ISBN 978-1-78238-732-9 hardback
ISBN 978-1-78238-733-6 ebook

For my mother,
my sisters,
my daughters
and you

Contents

ILLUSTRATIONS

Preface

I have previously explored other reproductive technologies in Thailand (namely contraception and abortion) and in particular the complexities they pose for women as they become intertwined with different political and personal circumstances. Unlike my previous work in Thailand, in this study I was working with urban elites, not subaltern villagers. At times I found this both uncomfortable and provoking and it caused me to reflect upon the privilege of my own position while underlining the fact that in many parts of the world, access to health care and the right to reproduce is limited to those with the money to pursue it. I do not posit any reproductive technology to be intrinsically negative for women nor inherently positive, and this ambivalence is evident in this book. Rather, I am interested in how choices present themselves to women in different times, places and contexts and how women and men negotiate these choices. I respect the 'moral pioneers' willing to engage in these life experiments, the patients and medical staff who participate in complex relationships with each other and the technologies. I am witness to the fractured identities, abusive treatments, failures, inequities and exploitation as well as the joys, excitement and determination involved in assisted reproduction. I both admire the sheer technical skill of clinicians and laboratory staff involved while questioning the effects upon women's subjectivities. I question easy assumptions entailed in words like 'choice', while noting that access to assisted reproductive technologies is fundamental to people's ability and right to choose to reproduce and form the families they desire. Across this book I hope to tease apart some of these complexities while acknowledging that they can never be resolved. Although I have not personally been a patient, I hope my own reproductive history, my experience of desired maternity, three pregnancies and reproductive loss grants me some empathy towards the couples whose words and experiences form the core of this book. The ethnographic enterprise to translate and present worlds from outside one's own culture necessarily complicates this view. All mistakes are mine, and I hope this book reflects my curiosity, empathy and respect for my informants as I consider their experiences.

ACKNOWLEDGEMENTS

A number of people contributed to this book. Foremost I wish to thank the anonymous doctors, clinic staff and in particular the patients of the two public and three private clinics who facilitated and participated in this study. I wish to thank Professor Roungsil Chaovaratana, head of the Infertility Clinic, Siriraj Hospital, for his support, and Dr Amara Soonthorndhada and the Institute for Population and Social Research, Mahidol University, especially for support as a visiting scholar during this research. I also wish to thank Professor Pramuan Virutamasen from Chulalongkorn Hospital for his time and support. I also thank Professor Kamheang Chaturachinda and Ms Nongluk Boonthai of the Women's Health and Reproductive Rights Foundation of Thailand for their continued assistance and support. I thank the Asia Research Institute, National University of Singapore, for a senior visiting fellowship that allowed me the time to write this study together.

I particularly wish to thank my friend and colleague Dr Parisa Rungruang, who worked as a research assistant during this project, Khun Jarucha Chotemanee for the translation of some of the interviews, and Kathleen Nolan and Dr Rachel Canaway for their assistance in the editing and formatting of the final manuscript.

A draft version of chapter 4 appeared as a paper within the Asian Research Institute Working paper series No. 182, April 2012, National University of Singapore. Parts of chapter 8 have previously appeared in the journal *Gender, Technology and Development,* 2014, volume 18, 1: 9–31. Ethical clearance to conduct the project was received from the University of Melbourne Human Research Ethics Committee (HREC 060504X. 2), the Faculty of Medicine, Mahidol University (016/2550) and clearances obtained through all participating hospitals and clinics and the National Research Council of Thailand (No. 0002. 3/2069). All names of informants and participating clinics remain anonymous and pseudonyms are used throughout this report and all publications. The research was funded by the Australian government through the Australian Research Council Discovery Project 'Infertility, IVF and reproductive tourism in Thailand and the region' and an ARC Future Fellowship. I wish to thank my colleagues at Monash University, and in particular Professor Lenore Manderson for her friendship, support and mentoring during the writing of this manuscript. Finally, I wish to thank my family: my husband, reader and colleague, Dr Bruce Missingham, and our daughters, Claire and Rachel, for accompanying me through fieldwork, sustaining me and teaching me the privilege and joys of mothering.

Notes on Language and Transliteration

Transcription of the Thai words used throughout this text follow the transcription system below. Under this system, tones and long vowels are not indicated. Exceptions to this system include place names, personal names and authors' names where the transcription system follows that customarily used. For consistency in the list of references, Thai authors are listed by their last names but their first names are indicated where available.

Thai Vowels

Phonetic symbol	*Thai symbol*	*Phonetic symbol*	*Thai symbol*
a	อะ, อั-, inherent	o	โอะ, inherent
a	อา	o	โอ
am	อำ	oi	โอย
ao	เอา	o	เอาะ
ao	อาว	o	ออ, inherent
ai	อัย, ใอ, ไอ	oi	ออย
ai	อาย	oe	เออะ
e	เอะ, เอ็-	oe	เออ, เอิ-
e	เอ	oei	เอย
ew	เอ็ว	u	อุ
ew	เอว	u	อู
ae	แอะ, แอ็-	ua	อว-, อัย, อัวะ
ae	แอ	uay	อวย
aew	แอว	ui	อุย
i	อิ	eu	อึ
i	อี	eu	อื-

ia	เอียะ, เอีย	eua	เอือะ, เอือ
iaw	เอียว	euay	เอือย
iw	อิว		
ru	ฤ, ฤๅ	lu	ฦ, ฦๅ

Thai Consonants Syllable-Initial Values

Phonetic Symbol	*Thai symbol*	*Phonetic Symbol*	*Thai symbol*
k	ก	ph	ผ, พ, ภ
kh	ข, ค, ฆ	f	ฝ, ฟ
ng	ง	m	ม
j	จ	y	ย, ญ
ch	ฉ, ช, ฌ	r	ร
d	ฎ, ด	l	ล, ฬ
t	ฏ, ต	w	ว
th	ฐ, ฑ, ฒ, ถ, ท, ธ	s	ซ, ศ, ษ, ส
n	ณ, น	h	ห, ฮ
b	บ	-	อ (glottal stop)
p	ป		

Thai Consonants Syllable-Final Values

Phonetic Symbol	*Thai Symbol*
k	ก, ข, ค, ฆ
ng	ง
t	จ, ฉ, ช, ซ, ฌ, ฎ, ฏ, ฐ, ฑ, ฒ, ด, ต, ถ, ท, ธ, ศ, ษ, ส
n	ญ, ณ, น, ล, ฬ
p	บ, ป, ผ, ฝ, พ, ฟ, ภ
m	ม
y or i	ย
w	ว

Abbreviations

ART	assisted reproductive technology
ESHRE	European Society for Human Reproduction and Embryology
GATS	general agreement on trades in services
GIFT	gamete intrafallopian transfer
GPO	government pharmaceutical organization
ICSI	intracytoplasmic sperm injection
IUI	intrauterine insemination
IVF	in vitro fertilization
OHSS	ovarian hyperstimulation syndrome
PESA	percutaneous epididymal sperm aspiration
PGD	preimplantation genetic diagnosis
PGS	preimplantation genetic screening
STD	sexually transmitted disease
TESE	testicular sperm extraction
ZIFT	zygote intrafallopian transfer

Introduction

Culture Mediums

We are in the hospital lift, leaving the clinic after a day of interviews. One of the women we had interviewed that morning is in the lift with us. During the interview she revealed that she had started bleeding and was in the clinic to get a blood test on the viability of her pregnancy. She was waiting for her results and while talking about it had become very upset, weeping quietly. We stopped the interview and comforted her and waited with her before she went in to see the doctor. The test was negative, another unsuccessful transfer. She had come alone to the clinic, so my Thai research assistant, Som, sat with her a while until she was calm.

We had been surprised to see her among the crowd of people in the lift, and cautiously smiled at her. She was looking intently at a young woman who was cradling a newborn baby in her arms. The baby was swaddled with a warm bonnet on its head and little gloves on its hands. She turned to the woman and asked, 'Is the baby *thammachaat* [natural]? Did you get it naturally?'

The woman looked quizzically at her, not sure what this odd question meant. She smiled in return.

'Is it a *dek lord kaew* [glass tube baby] or is it natural, did you get it naturally all by yourselves?' she asked.

'No, naturally, by ourselves', the young mother replied, a little uncomfortable at this intrusive question.

'Oh, you are clever', she admired sadly. The new mother smiled faintly and looked at the door.

This uncomfortable moment in the lift exemplifies the everyday tragedies endured by couples wanting children in Thailand who are undergoing assisted reproductive treatments. This book is about assisted reproductive technologies in Thailand, the people who use them and the industry that maintains their use. My aim in this book is to explore how assisted reproductive technologies have been introduced and incorporated into Thai understandings and practices surrounding reproduction. I provide insight into the particularities of assisted reproduction in Thailand and the history and use of assisted reproduction from the perspectives of patients and providers.

The term 'assisted reproductive technologies' refers to the range of biomedical technologies used in noncoital reproduction in which gametes are manipulated or embryos are created outside of the body. It includes techniques such as intrauterine insemination (IUI) through to high-tech in vitro fertilization (IVF) techniques and newer technologies such as preimplantation genetic diagnosis (PGD) of embryos before transfer to a woman's uterus, and intracytoplasmic sperm injection (ICSI) (see glossary for definitions). They are used to assist people who are involuntarily infertile to have children and form families. They can also be used for genetic screening when there is no medical diagnosis of infertility. There is a huge range of techniques that can be used in assisted reproduction. In this book I concentrate upon IVF techniques involving egg extraction, sperm collection and preparation and fertilization, including the use of ICSI. I also include the use of surrogates undergoing in vitro procedures to carry a pregnancy for another woman. I concentrate upon Thai users of these techniques. Although Thai clinics also provide assisted reproductive services for foreign couples, within this book I am interested only in how Thai users and providers approach reproduction through these technologies.

Assisted reproductive technologies have spread across the globe. They can be considered one example of the impact of global flows of technologies upon the experiences and understandings of our bodies. The Thai use of reproductive biotechnologies I present in this book is a case study of similar effects happening throughout the world, albeit with localized variations. An abundant anthropological literature now documents the uses and practices of these technologies in diverse settings.[1] They demonstrate how the intimacies of reproduction – the ways in which we form families and reproduce – are being profoundly impacted by the movement of technologies of assisted reproduction, the sharing of biomedical information and expertise, the production of new forms of knowledge about reproduction and the body, the growth of biosocial identities and the travel of patients, gametes and reproductive assistors (surrogates, ova and sperm donors) (see discussion in Inhorn and Birenbaum-Carmeli 2008).

Assisted Reproduction in Thailand

It is estimated that 10–15 per cent of Thai couples in the reproductive age range have infertility problems and that there are around 10 million infertile couples in Thailand (Boonkasemsanti et al. 2000, cited in Chiamchanya and Su-Angkawatin 2008). Since the first IVF baby was born at Chulalongkorn Hospital in 1987 (see chapter 1), assisted reproductive technologies have quickly spread throughout the country. All major public tertiary hospitals offer assisted reproductive technologies, but the majority of providers are in private hospitals or specialist clinics. According to the National Assisted Reproductive Technology (ART) registry of the Royal Thai College of Obstetricians and Gynaecologists, in 2010 there were thirty clinics licensed to provide assisted reproductive treatments in Thailand, evidence of the rapid global penetration of new reproductive technologies into Thailand. Three-quarters of these clinics are clustered in Bangkok while other centres are located in the major regional towns.

The assisted reproductive industry in Thailand is highly sophisticated with overall success rates comparable with those of overseas clinics. Results from the National ART registry found the average pregnancy rate for in vitro fertilization was 28.9 per cent per retrieval or 33.8 per cent per embryo transfer – comparable with clinics elsewhere (Vutyavanich et al. 2011). Their data confirmed the findings of overseas clinics that clinics with higher cycle volumes achieve significantly higher pregnancy rates than smaller clinics, probably due to differences in clinical or laboratory expertise.

The use of assisted reproductive technologies is associated with a risk of multiple pregnancies. Thai clinics have a multiple pregnancy rate of 11.4 per cent (Vutyavanich et al. 2011). Triplet or higher-order multiple pregnancies account for around 3 per cent of live births. The ART registry reports that elective single embryo transfer is not practiced in Thailand and that the driving force behind transfer of multiple embryos is the fact that the cost of cycles is borne by the infertile couple.

Assisted reproductive technologies advance rapidly with consequent shifts in techniques offered at clinics. For example, over a seven-year period the more invasive gamete (GIFT) and zygote intrafallopian transfer (ZIFT) techniques decreased from 10.6 per cent of all fresh cycles in 2001 to only 1 per cent in 2007 as advances in embryo culture techniques have improved the success rates from IVF (Vutyavanich et al. 2011). As a technology offering the possibility for infertile men to become biological fathers, ICSI has become increasingly popular. By 2007 ICSI accounted for 63 per cent of all cycles undertaken in Thailand, with some clinics routinely performing ICSI regardless of sperm quality, despite (or perhaps because of) its higher cost and longer laboratory time required and the fact that it has not been shown to increase success rates in couples with nonmale infertility. The advent of PGD and preimplantation genetic screening (PGS) is likewise rapidly expanding in Thailand. By 2006, ten centres were offering PGS (many for nonmedical sex selection) and four centres were offering PGD (primarily for thalassemia) (Vutyavanich et al. 2011).

The introduction of high-tech conception comes at a time of increased medicalization of birthing and wide public acceptance of technological interventions. As I witnessed in the early 1990s (Whittaker 1999) hospital-based birthing has replaced older styles of birthing formerly practiced at home with birth attendants or midwives. This 'birthing transition' (Haora 2013) is characterized by a high level of interventions such as episiotomies and caesarean sections (with a rate over 50 per cent in private hospitals since 1996), well over the World Health Organization's (WHO) recommended rate of 10–15 per cent (Chanrachakul et al. 2000). Although critics within Thailand view the current status of birthing as overmedicalized (Tangcharoensathien et al. 2002) as will be seen later in this book, caesarean births are widely believed to be safer and the dominance of technologized births reflects the pre-eminence, prestige and trust placed in biomedicine within Thai society. Faith in 'modern' technology and willingness to accept biomedical interventions in reproduction has also characterized the Thai public's approaches to assisted reproduction.

Access to Assisted Reproduction

One issue that forms a subtext to this study is the differential access to assisted reproductive treatments. In developing countries, assisted reproductive treatments remain inaccessible for most couples experiencing infertility. Only 48 out of 191 member states of the World Health Organization have IVF facilities (Inhorn 2009; Akande 2008). There is a high demand for biomedical interventions with an estimated 56 per cent of infertile couples worldwide seeking some form of care (Boivin et al. 2007). Globally, it is estimated that less than 20 per cent of people requiring in vitro fertilization and associated technologies are actually using it, even in developed countries (Vayena et al. 2009). In vitro fertilization costs are approximately 50 per cent higher than the yearly annual income per capita of citizens in many developing countries, including India, Indonesia, China and Malaysia (Ombelet et al. 2008; Vayena et al. 2009). In 2001 the WHO called for innovative approaches such as the development of low-cost ART for low resource settings (Vayena et al. 2009); yet at the same time that those strategies are being implemented to improve access in developing countries, a number of those countries, including Thailand, are now involved in a global ART trade, while their local populations still struggle to afford access to these same technologies. Helena Ragoné and France Winddance Twine (2000: 6) note that the privileging of elites in this fashion 'can be considered neo-eugenic to the extent that they privilege the reproduction of educated and upper-class women over that of other women'. This poses a new example of 'stratified reproduction' (Ginsburg and Rapp 1991) whereby inequalities empower certain categories of people to reproduce and nurture, but disempower others.

Most people who would benefit from these technologies in Thailand are unable to access them. Terapron Vutyavanich et al. (2011) estimate that given the Thai population of 65 million, the total number of IVF cycles required annually to meet need would be 97,605 cycles. However, fewer than 4,500 cycles were undertaken in Thailand in 2007, less than 5 per cent 'optimal' IVF utilization. As the Thai national health policy and private health insurance makes no provisions to cover infertility treatment, the cost of treatment is borne by patients.

The majority of women and men who I met through this research are middle class to upper class elites (see appendix). Most have the financial resources to undertake 'high-tech' treatments. As such, this book provides only a partial view of how people deal with infertility in Thailand. It needs to be remembered that in Thailand in the absence of publically funded IVF, the vast majority of peasant farmers cannot afford access to IVF and so are only ever offered lower-cost alternatives such as IUI. This study included only a few women from lower socioeconomic status. Poorer women face enormous pressures for their IVF treatment to succeed as they are gambling with their financial security. The difference between public and private treatment lies in costs from an average of US $2,900 per cycle in government hospitals to US $5,800 or more per cycle in private centres (Vutyavanich et al. 2011). Even among middle class patients, repeated cycles of IVF to produce a child cause considerable financial pain. Within public hospitals, doctors frequently remarked to me that they judge people's ability to pay and will only offer affordable treatments according to their assessments of what a couple can pay, so as not to set up unattainable expectations. The result is that IVF clinics have become exclusive – run by a handful of elite doctors catering to wealthy patients.

The differential access to assisted reproductive treatment continues despite the incorporation of a broader concept of reproductive health in Thai health policies. In July 1997 the Thai government released a National Reproductive Health Policy Statement reinforcing that 'All Thai citizens at all ages must have good reproductive health throughout their entire lives' (cited in UNFPA 2005: 14). This has coincided with policies encouraging integrated reproductive health services, not just family planning, promising greater inclusivity and quality of care and catering to the needs of marginalized groups. These include programs in adolescent health, sex education, post-abortion care, premarital counselling, women's health counselling and prevention of mother-to-child transmission of HIV, prevention and treatment of reproductive tract infections and malignancy, infertility and post-reproductive care (UNFPA 2005). However, despite the recognition of infertility as a reproductive health issue, there is no state funding of infertility treatments other than the most basic interventions.

The lack of treatment options for poorer couples was evident during fieldwork I undertook in the 1990s in a public hospital outpatients gynaecology clinic in the northeast of Thailand. I recall one woman around twenty-seven years of age presented seeking treatment for infertility. She was a peasant farmer from a nearby village. After an examination and history taking, the gynaecologist prescribed some tablets in the hope that they may assist her. As she left the room he turned to me and said, 'Really I feel bad when I see cases like her. She is a good candidate for IVF, it would really help her. But I know she can't afford it, so I don't even mention it to her.'

Familial adoption remains a common strategy for poorer infertile couples. This involves an infertile couple raising a child from a relative who has a large number of children. They are referred to as the *'phor mae liang'*, or nurturing parents of the child. As will be discussed later in this book, among the urban couples interviewed for this study, such forms of familial adoption are considered preferable to adoption of a child of unknown heritage. However, such arrangements are becoming less common as the possibility of genetic relatedness is pursued through assisted reproduction.

Religious Views of Assisted Reproduction

Local moral worlds, religious and ethical orders can be challenged by assisted reproduction. Different religious traditions define and regulate the use of these technologies variously.[2] But religious opinions do not necessarily govern people's actions; for example, the denunciation of assisted reproduction by the Roman Catholic Church does not prevent the practice of these technologies throughout most countries with majority Catholic populations (Roberts 2006). The majority of Thais are Theravadan Buddhist and Buddhist notions of *bun* and *bap* (meritorious acts and demerit) reincarnation and the importance of *kam* (karma) influencing the life course inform people's everyday actions.

There is no single authoritative Buddhist position on assisted reproduction in Thailand. When asked, local Buddhist commentators tend to support the use of assisted reproduction as a meritorious act undertaken for nonselfish reasons facilitating the rebirth of another life force. However, the status of the embryo poses particular ethical issues; in particular the question of what happens to excess embryos, their manipulation, disposal or storage, donation or use in research. Leading Buddhist bioethicist Pinit Ratanakul notes that Buddhism interprets life as beginning with conception:

> Thai Buddhist monks and lay people alike believe in the uniqueness and preciousness of human life irrespective of the stages of its development.... Human life begins at the very moment of fertilization with the infusion of the *gandhabba*, the individual karmic life-force, into the womb. Even though human life manifests in a minute form, called *kalala* in Buddhist terminology, it is still precious, and its destruction is a transgression of the Buddhist precept against killing. (Ratanakul 1999: 56)

In Thailand, questions over the disposition of embryos remain unresolved in many clinics, many are still developing their protocols for their patients' decision making; reluctance to destroy embryos makes some clinics line their corridors with storage containers. Advances in reproductive genetics and the increasing use of tests such as preimplantation genetic diagnosis, allowing for the early detection and selection of genetic disorders and sex selection, challenge notions of the sanctity of life in its early stages, allowing for the culling of genetically imperfect embryos or embryos of the undesirable sex. Damien Keown (1995: 135) suggests that because of the destruction of embryos involved, many of the practices of assisted reproduction would be considered undesirable from a Buddhist ethical position. Similarly, it is noted that in the United States, couples decisions over disposition of embryos are fraught and often unresolved (Nachtigall et al. 2005); in contrast, in India it is suggested that donations of spare embryos towards stem cell research are seen as altruistic (Bharadwaj 2009) fuelling a human embryonic stem cell industry.

Legal Status of Assisted Reproduction in Thailand

This study comes at a time of legal change which has profound ramifications for the practices of assisted reproduction in Thailand. Until 2010 assisted reproduction was largely unregulated in Thailand. Thailand had no specific law on assisted reproductive technologies. The Thai Medical Council introduced professional guidelines in 1997 and 2001 (Announcements 1/2540 and 21/2544) for assisted reproductive technologies. These guidelines were minimal, prescribing that that the Royal Thai College of Obstetricians and Gynaecologists was responsible for the supervision and administration of assisted reproductive technologies and that each centre offering assisted reproductive technologies is required to have an ethics committee of at least three staff members and collect a husband and wife's written consent for all procedures (Virutamasen et al. 2001). These guidelines had no legislative force. As will be described in the next chapter, with increasing use of these technologies and a growing number of legal cases involving its use pressure grew for legislation. It was not until 11 May 2010 that the Thai cabinet approved draft legislation of the 'Pregnancy by Medically Assisted Reproductive Technology Act' bill number 167/2553 (Adams 2010).[3]

As will be described later, a series of highly publicized incidents in Thailand from 2011–2014, revealed a range of practices within clinics, including commercial international surrogacy and ova donation that contravened the spirit if not the letter of regulations in Thailand. These included the case of Baby Gammy, a child with Down's syndrome allegedly abandoned in Thailand by his Australian intended parents (and biological father) to be cared for by his gestational surrogate while his twin sister was taken to Australia (Whiteman 2014, Murdoch 2014). On 22 July 2014, the military government, the National Peace and Order Council announced a review of all 12 Thai IVF clinics involved in surrogacy cases believed to be possibly involved in breaches of the Thai Medical Council guidelines and not certified by the Royal College of Obstetricians. At the time of writing the bill had been approved by the current military government, the National Council for Peace and Order (NCPO), and passed by the National Legislative Assembly for endorsement (Ruangdit and Intathep, 2014). It is expected that in 2015 the bill will pass further reading by the Senate and will then be passed to His Majesty the King of Thailand for assent then promulgation in Royal Gazette to become law.

This act strictly regulates the use of assisted reproductive technologies in Thailand and clarifies the legal status of children born through these technologies. The draft endorses the Medical Council's regulations and sets out punishments for medical professionals breaching the provisions. The draft law covers the criteria for the donation of eggs or sperm, their storage and the use of ART. It prohibits the use of the egg or sperm of donors who have died without leaving written consent. Preimplantation genetic diagnosis is allowed for medical reasons but not for the purpose of gender selection (Article 17)[4] clearly defining sex selection for social reasons as unethical and illegal.

Significantly, the draft legislation clarifies the legal status of children and intended parents and provides certain protections for surrogates. It specifically outlaws commercial ova donation and commercial surrogacy arrangements (see chapter 9). It limits surrogacy to procedures using the ova and sperm of a heterosexual married couple, or using the ova or sperm of either a husband or wife paired with the sperm or egg of another donor. A surrogate must have had a child before and if married must have the permission of her husband before undergoing surrogacy. The draft law authorizes the Medical Council to set the criteria, methods and financial conditions for the care of surrogate mothers before, during and after the pregnancy.

The legislation also reverses the uterocentric legal definition of motherhood which prevailed in Thailand. Until 2015 the legal mother of a child was the woman who gave birth to the child. Section 1546 of the Thai Civil and Commercial Code provides[5]: 'A child born of a woman who is not married to a man is deemed to be the legitimate child of the woman.' The consequence of this code provision has been that intended parents needed to adopt any child produced through a surrogacy arrangement. Also, an intended father had no rights over a child produced through surrogacy even if he was the biological father of the child, unless various legal procedures were undertaken to grant him those rights. Under this legislation the commissioning parents are recognized as the legal parents of the child. The law also precludes the egg donor from any parenting rights. The Juvenile and Family Court will be authorized to judge paternity cases for children born through assisted reproduction and protect the legal rights and status of children.

Studying Thai In Vitro

My aim in this book is to capture the current practices, understandings and experiences of Thai couples undergoing assisted reproductive treatment. This book is based upon a multisite research project in one public and three private clinics in Bangkok across eight months in 2007–2008.[6] A total of thirty-one women, thirteen men and six staff were interviewed (see appendix).

A number of the people interviewed were followed up over time with repeat interviews and telephone follow-ups. In addition, observations were undertaken at the clinics, and at various shrines and sacred places associated with infertility. To place the Thai study within the broader sociopolitical context I also undertook a search of the media and popular press for the popular discursive context of infertility and assisted conception services in Thailand as well as a systematic collection of Thai language websites/blogs and web boards aimed at infertile people. This allowed me to link the private experiences of men and women to the representations of infertility and reproductive technologies in the media, religious socialization and public policy. The study is also grounded in my previous long-term field experience working in Thailand that included an ethnography on rural women's reproductive health, and studies of other reproductive technologies such as contraception and abortion (Whittaker 2000, 2002b, 2004).

Participants in this study were recruited through the clinics that informed potential participants who were then given an information statement explaining the research. If they agreed to be interviewed they would then meet my Thai colleague Dr Parisa Rungruang (Som), who assisted me throughout data collection, and myself. Following written permission, all interviews were taped and later transcribed in Thai and translated into English by Thai research assistants and myself. Only one participant refused the use of a tape recorder. The interviews were semi-structured with certain demographic and personal information collected from all participants but then followed by open-ended questions, allowing the interviewee freedom to give their stories and express what they felt was important. Interviews usually took place either at the clinic following or before a regular scheduled appointment at a private location within the clinic, or at a place determined by the patient. Similar studies in other settings have noted that participants often appreciate the opportunity interviews give for an outsider to share and appreciate their stories, and this was our experience in both this research and previous research on similarly sensitive matters (see Inhorn 2004a).

Given the fact that recruitment took place within a clinical context, care was taken to ensure that distressed patients or those not medically fit to be interviewed were excluded from participation. Doctors and clinical staff were not aware of which of their patients actually accepted to participate in the study. No real names of patients, staff or clinics are used in this book to help protect the identities of participants. Ethical permission was obtained from my university human ethics committee as well as participating clinics and the National Research Council of Thailand.[7]

Approaches in this Book

My previous work in Thailand has been concerned with situating the ethnographic detail of reproductive health issues within the broader social, cultural and political economic context. Likewise, in this book I continue my ongoing interest in the social and moral meanings of bodies and health and the 'politics of reproduction' (Ginsburg and Rapp 1991) – the political and economic constraints which structure reproductive decisions. This is combined with a desire to capture the cultural flows, in particular the flows of people, technologies and imaginaries within globalized reproductive and productive spaces. My analysis is grounded in the data I collected and draws selectively upon both structural and poststructural social theories (Foucault and Deleuze 1977). As such the book is an attempt to interlace an ethnography of IVF users with insights on the ways in which the technologies themselves influence behaviours from science and technology studies.

Assisted Reproduction as an Assemblage

I utilize the concept of assemblage to characterize the multiple dimensions of assisted reproduction. The concept of assemblage captures configurations that emerge from shifting social relationships among diverse things, sites and people (Deleuze and Guattari 2003; DeLanda 2002; Marcus and Saka 2006). Andrew Pickering (1992) for example uses the term 'heterogenous assemblages' to describe the contingent coming together of technologies and humans to create new knowledge and practices. Paul Rabinow (2003) speaks of his primary research object as assemblages, 'the distinctive type of experimental matrix of heterogenous elements, techniques, and concepts'. This notion of assemblages has since been applied by anthropologists such as Aihwa Ong and Stephen Collier (2005) to explore the ensembles of heterogeneous elements through which to reflect upon the human impact of contemporary technoscientific issues. They define 'global assemblages' as 'how global forms interact with other elements, occupying a common field in contingent, uneasy, unstable interrelationships.... As a composite concept, the term "global assemblage" suggests inherent tensions: global implies broadly encompassing, seamless, and mobile; assemblage implies heterogeneous, contingent, unstable, partial, and situated' (Ong and Collier 2005: 12).

Within this book, I use 'global assemblage' to assist in capturing the heterogeneous relations, techniques and concepts inherent in practices of assisted reproduction. How we constitute reproduction itself is being reimagined – it is not just a capacity of sexed bodies, but is rendered through an assemblage of fusing cells, bodies, practices, pharmaceuticals, technology, capital, economics, politics, law, trade, travel and nations. This book describes a local instantiation of this assemblage; how it is deeply entangled in larger transnational circulations and actively shaped by structural inequalities; and yet takes on local inflections. As an anthropologist I am interested in considering how such technological assemblages are constituted and enacted in their particularities – the phenomenological effects and affects of the technologies, bodies, processes and interventions.

Globalization and the Dissemination and Localization of Technologies

The starting point for this book then is the concept of assisted reproductive technologies as globalized technologies. Assisted reproduction is an enterprise reflecting the 'the global penetration of modern institutions into the tissue of day-to-day life' (Ong and Collier 2005: 8). In the same way as the introduction of contraceptive technologies across the world provoked a range of social and moral sensitivities, resistances and alliances, so too the introduction of new reproductive technologies raises questions about how local sociocultural, economic and political considerations shape how technologies are both offered to and received across different cultural settings, or what Arjun Appadurai (1996) has termed the 'localization' of technologies. Across the pages of this book there is a constant interplay between localized manifestations and global forms. As Ong and Collier (2005: 11) note, technoscience is exemplary of global forms – able to assimilate itself to new environments, move across diverse social and cultural situations and be recontextualized and reterritorrialized. As practices and technologies dealing intimately with bodies, life, notions of kinship, ethical regimes, social and biological generation and gendered identities; assisted reproduction is a case study in how forms of technoscience take on local inflections and are transmuted into new forms which may themselves take on global significance. One contribution of this book is to provide a further ethnographically informed example to our growing understanding of how these technologies are deployed, practiced, consumed and experienced.

Although there are differences in the ways in which globalization is conceptualized, it is generally agreed that we live in a time of intensified economic, informational and communication linkages and networks on a scale and pace hitherto not experienced. Globalization is also characterized by increased flows in technologies, such as transport and information technologies, environmental engineering and biotechnologies. The increased global flows of information, media forms, Internet, education institutions, religious groups and political parties are also leading to cognitive changes in how we see ourselves and the world around us – a 'new role for the imagination in social life' (Appadurai 1996: 31). For Appadurai these new imaginaries are: 'a form of negotiation between sites of agency (individuals) and globally defined fields of possibility' (1996: 31). Global technologies such as assisted reproduction are expanding our definitions of families and social life with new possibilities. Writing of the global spread of assisted reproductive technologies, Frank van Balen and Marcia Inhorn (2002: 27) suggest, 'The availability of NRTs [new reproductive technologies] in disparate global sites may create new possibilities, new social imaginaries, and new arenas of cultural production, as well as new contradictions, new dilemmas of agency and new regimes of control.'

Another way of conceptualizing the multiple dimensions of global phenomena, has been through metaphors of landscapes. With regard to reproductive technologies and most particularly the trade in gametes and reproductive travel, Inhorn (2011) has taken up Appadurai's (1996: 31) conceptualization of five 'scapes' – the '-scape' suffix suggesting both the irregularities of these landscapes but also the ways in which they are 'deeply perspectival constructs' dependent upon who is observing.[8] She suggests the concept of a 'reproscape' of moving biological substances and body parts. This 'meta-scape' involves circulating reproductive technologies and flows of reproductive actors and gametes within a large-scale industry in which images and ideas about reproduction and tourism destinations and reproductive imaginaries abound. Unlike Appadurai's conceptualization of 'scapes', Inhorn draws attention to how this reproscape is highly gendered, and stratifies risk. This reproscape is formed through localized layers of meanings and histories, uneven fissures stratify access across class and ethnicity, technological practices are metamorphosed through pressures from global capital as patients, clinicians, embryos and gametes traverse its spaces. Analytically, the concept of a reproscape is very similar to that of an assemblage, although it highlights the importance of place, spatial movement and perspective. One difficulty is that the landscape metaphor it evokes is perhaps more static than intended and less able to capture the shifting contingencies that occur in everyday practices of health, illness and technological use.

This Book

The book starts with an historical account of IVF in Thailand, from the first test tube baby in 1987 through to present controversies. Based upon extensive research in Thai-language newspapers and other media, as well as interviews with some of the key clinicians involved, I explore the shifting constructions of assisted reproductive technologies in the media and the social meanings attached to them. The Thai public has been quick to embrace assisted reproduction. Since the birth of the first Thai *dek lord kaew* (glass tube baby), assisted reproductive technologies have generally been celebrated. Possibly because assisted reproductive technologies were not publicly funded, they have been allowed to proliferate with little state intervention. The last thirty years have seen the rapid expansion of assisted reproductive technologies and expertise across the country. Medically assisted reproductive technologies such as IVF have quickly become associated with positive imagery of science, modernity, high technology and strong maternal desire. As will be seen throughout this book, they have become associated with the pursuit of an ideal family form – a small, upper middle class heterosexual family.

Margaret Lock (1998) suggests that 'if the application of reproductive technologies do not coincide rather closely with widely shared societal values, they may well be judged as disruptive to the moral order, no matter how well packaged and promoted'. Similarly, technologies that do fit in with shared social values become 'naturalized' (Lock and Kaufert 1998) as supporting the moral order and become an unquestioned part of people's reproductive lives. Assisted technologies fit well the values of the small Thai family and Thai women as responsible mothers validated by the state.

This book then moves onto considering the experience of infertility in Thai society and the multiple resorts to care undertaken by the infertile couples of this study. Chapter 2 describes understandings of infertility and the stigma associated with it for women and men. As I explain, children are highly valued in Thailand and the normative expectation is that a couple will start a family shortly after marriage. Couples without children in this study describe themselves as 'incomplete' in their marriage but also as individuals for failing to fulfil gendered expectations. Chapter 3 explores the 'sacred geography' of fertility in Thailand, the shrines and sacred places utilized by infertile couples in their attempts to seek care and treatment. It introduces another subtext of this book – the enchantment of assisted reproduction. Emblematic of the social nature of technologies is the ways in which their use and practice reveals a range of rituals, social meanings and contingencies. In this book I utilize the notion of enchantment as a means to illustrate this social and spiritual relationship with/in technologies. I show how, far from being strictly scientific, Thai patients and clinicians approach assisted reproduction with a degree of faith and mystery, the efficacy of which is defined as much by karma as laboratory results.

I consider the ways in which religious belief continues to play an important role in reproduction in Thailand, even within a select population committed to 'high-tech' interventions to cure their infertility. The array of Buddhist, Brahman, Taoist and Hindu religious sites, natural and ancestral spirits and royal spirits, reflects the diversity and hybridity of Thai religious belief and practice. I argue that many of the shrines have particular gendered significance for women in their pursuit of children – a means to intervene in the supernatural world without the mediation of (male) monks. They represent further examples of the intersection between the sacred and the ordinary, religion and magic in Thai society.

Such pilgrimages in the spiritual realm have their own parallels in treatment seeking within the biomedical realm. Both involve syncretic care seeking at multiple sites, both are enveloped by a sense of enchantment and appeal to various sources of authority. In Thailand infertile couples seek intervention from gods and spirits in conjunction with high-tech treatments. Faith and karmic fortune is believed fundamental to the efficacy of both. As I then describe in chapter 4, the very rituals and interventions of the clinics, the offerings and discipline involved find its parallels in the shrines and sacred places visited for spiritual interventions.

Chapter 4 begins an exploration of the experiences of patients in infertility clinics using assisted reproductive technologies, primarily IVF procedures. I explore the medicalization of patients and its effects. It documents the experiences of patients of the liminal space of the clinic and the process of becoming a patient, undergoing interventions and cycles, their failures and successes. Charis Thompson (2005) describes the process of assisted reproduction as one of 'ontological choreography' – the 'coordination of the technical, scientific, kinship, gender, emotional, legal, political and financial aspects of ART clinics: the coming together of things generally considered parts of different ontological orders'. This process involves the 'grafting of parts and calibrating of time' (2005), the normalization of medical procedures, socialization of patients and naturalization of the technologies.

Within the clinic similar processes of intense medicalization can be observed. Assisted reproduction involves the monitoring, surveillance and creation of data about infertile women and men. The focus upon and abstraction of women and men's bodies and embryonic bodies, and fetishization of sophisticated machinery all operate within these settings. I note how these processes cast their own enchantment as practices become ritualized, patients bodies are blamed for failures and clinicians act as mediators to the mysteries of conception.

However, it is simplistic to suggest that the unequal power relations and politics embedded within reproductive technologies are fixed and unalterable. Rather, the effects can be disempowering but also productive – actively chosen, even demanded by the participants. As seen throughout this chapter, patients may not only endure but embrace the reductive view of their bodies and actively pursue and participate in the monitoring of body processes. They may subscribe deeply to an imagined future and the promise held by technology, to the detriment of their careers, social relations and against the advice of their doctors.

In chapter 5 I present insights into the 'clinical ensemble'; the various actors involved in infertility treatment, providing views from clinicians, nurse counsellors and embryologists about their work. Staff describe themselves as having a special vocation to help patients form families and create life. Yet their views of their service orientation are not always shared by their patients. Thai patients generally defer to their doctor's advice and rarely challenge their opinions despite the poor communication, rushed consultations and lack of empathy some patients experience. Patients who become pregnant speak in glowing terms of their medical staff, yet the experience of failed cycles strains their trust in their doctors and 'shopping around' for doctors is common. Differences in the level of service available in private clinics compared to public clinics are commented upon by patients, as are accusations of profiteering as patients experience levels of intervention and expense.

This book draws upon a heritage of feminist studies of reproduction concerned with gender-based inequalities and discrimination, practices of stratification, agency and resistance, which describe biomedical science as a location of masculinist power applied to women's bodies. But in this book I present a more nuanced view of women's agency within medical treatment. In chapter 6 I describe the ways in which some women consciously make patriarchal bargains in their use of these technologies – undertaking treatment to secure their relationships, fulfil their obligations to the family lineage and ensure their economic future. The very act of undertaking treatment is used to demonstrate their commitment to their relationships. Women and men in this study are constantly involved in a project of negotiating reproductive outcomes for themselves consonant with what is both expected of them, but also to satisfy their own aspirations. Where exactly the boundaries and limits to agency and expectation lie and how these are worked out by various women and men is only illuminated through ethnographic inquiry.

In chapter 7 I explore the interface of medically assisted reproduction and the Internet and the resultant new biological knowledge, social identities and forms of collective identity making. Through an exploration of the Thai-language *'Love Clinic'* (*Clinicrak*) chat room and other similar sites used by people undergoing treatment with assisted reproductive technologies, I explore how cyberspace allows forms of association between people with fertility difficulties unavailable in other spaces. I concentrate upon how the Internet offers a form of virtual community for people for whom no other forums for sociality exists. I argue that these forms of identity and biosociality (Rabinow 1996) involve dialogue between older and newer forms of identity construction and understandings of infertility, redefining the meanings and practices of these groups. Finally, this chapter explores the limits of the relationship between such forms of biosociality and citizenship and why these particular communities lack the transformative power evident for other biosocial groupings in Thai society.

Men's experiences of assisted reproduction are often ignored and needs overlooked (Inhorn 2002, 2004b, 2006a; Carmeli and Birenbaum-Carmeli 1994). Chapter 8 explores how Thai men's experiences of assisted reproduction and men's actions are also influenced by patriarchal norms and expectations. Within Thailand, male infertility remains deeply stigmatized due to insinuations of impotence and emasculation. Although men were reticent about their experiences, they gave insights into the social pressures to father a child, the imperative to have a biological child and dislike of donor sperm or adoption, their embarrassment at having to perform masturbation on a schedule to provide sperm samples, the pain of testicular surgeries. New technologies such as ICSI have revolutionized the treatment of male infertility, but themselves carry gendered implications as men and women are compelled to try this new technology.

Although the effects of these technologies upon notions of motherhood and kinship have been discussed within Western settings (Becker 2000; Franklin 1997; Ragoné 1994; Thompson 2005), less is understood about how other cultural understandings of kinship may be affected. Surrogacy and ova donation are deconstructing motherhood into genetic, birth, adoptive and surrogate maternities and the potential for a child to have three biological mothers (Sandelowski 1993). Angela Davis (1998) speaks of the creation of 'alienated and fragmented maternities'. Chapter 9 examines surrogacy through a case study of Ying, a commissioning parent talking about her relationship with her surrogate. Ying has a long history of infertility treatment, and we learn of her experience and emotions during repeated attempts at using IVF, a donor ova and surrogacy. This chapter highlights the complexities of the relationship between an intended parent and surrogate. Her narrative reveals insidious power differentials between surrogate and intended parent. This is exacerbated by the financial and proprietal rights implied over the surrogate's body. The threat surrogacy poses for Thai sensibilities and notions of motherhood is clear in the continued secrecy and ambiguity involved in surrogacy arrangements in Thailand, yet even surrogacy is being increasingly accepted and naturalized – forthcoming legislation reversing the traditional uterocentric notion of a mother as the one who gives birth in favour of commissioning parents marks a turning point in Thai conceptions of maternity and kinship. The clear restrictions contained in this legislation against gay and single-parent use of assisted reproductive technologies however reasserts a married heteronormative definition of a Thai family against the subversive potential of assisted reproductive technologies for the creation of new family forms.

Conclusions

I understand these technologies to both recreate and transform class, gender and ethnic divisions in Thai society through the stratification and privileging of certain types of people to reproduce. However, it would be a mistake for this book to equate what is presented merely to stories of exploitation; rather, I hope the book is read as the problematic striving, the experimentation with technoscientific practices that can enhance and enable life but in doing so are also subject to contradictions and corruptions. Throughout this book there are encounters with the contradictory effects of these quests—patriarchal bargains, the entrenchment of patriarchal power relations, the commodification and dissection of the reproductive body into parts at the same time as women and men and medical staff describe the technology in terms of hope, life, their agency, choice and ardent desires to achieve parenthood.

Notes

1. These include studies of assisted reproductive technologies and infertility in: Vietnam (Pashigan 2002, 2009), China (Handwerker 2002), Sri Lanka (Dissanayake, Simpson and Jayasekara 2002; Simpson, Dissanayake and Jayasekara 2005), India (Bharadwaj 2009; Pande 2010, 2011; Riessman 2000, 2002), Iran (Tremayne 2009), Egypt (Inhorn 1994, 1996, 2003a, 2003b), Israel (Birenbaum-Carmeli 2007; Kahn 2000; Nahman 2011), Greece (Paxson 2003, 2006), Italy (Bonaccorso 2009), Argentina (Raspberry 2009) and Ecuador (Roberts 2009).
2. See discussion in van Balen 2009. Among Sunni Muslims, gamete donation and surrogacy have been religiously proscribed, however Shia Muslim fatwas in Iran and Lebanon facilitate third-party donations in these

countries (Inhorn 2006b; Tremayne 2006, 2009). In Israel assisted reproduction is state subsidized and religiously condoned, with rabbinical law proving flexible to accommodate the full range of assisted technologies, surrogacy and gamete donations (Kahn 2000, 2006; Birenbaum-Carmeli and Inhorn 2009; Nahman 2006).

3. See Thailand, Council of State. 2010. *Rangphrachabun natikhumkhrongdek thi kert doi asai teknoloyi kan jaloernphan thangkanphaet* (Civil Decree no. 167/2553), http://web.krisdika.go.th/data/news/news10866.pdf (accessed 20 May 2014); and Nanthida Puangthong's article, 2010, 'New Draft Law to Protect Surrogate Mothers, Offspring', *The Nation*, http://www.nationmultimedia.com/home/2010/05/12/national/New-draft-law-to-protect-surrogate-mothers-offspri-30129064.html (accessed 20 May 2014).
4. Translation provided by Parisa Rungruang.
5. Sandhikshetrin, Kamol. 2008. *The Civil and Commercial Code Books I-VI and Glossary*, 7th ed. Bangkok: Nitibannakan. http://en.wikisource.org/wiki/Civil_and_Commercial_Code/Current_Version/Book_5 (accessed 20 May 2014).
6. As Inhorn (2004a) has noted, it is difficult to gain permission to work within clinics and I am very grateful to those clinicians who gave me access and facilitated my access to other clinics through their former students. This was partly achieved through introductions from contacts made through my previous work in Thailand and by my very bad karaoke-singing effort at a workshop held in Chiang Rai with members of the Royal Thai College of Obstetrics and Gynaecology.
7. As with any study, this one has a number of limitations. Firstly, as a clinic-based study it only includes those people already undergoing assisted reproductive treatment. I make no claims of generalizability. As a study of current patients, it does not include the voices of people who may have decided not to utilize these technologies, nor those who may have tried but then decided to cease treatment. As such, the people in this book probably have more positive views of the technologies than others. As I was recruiting within the clinics, my sample also does not include those who were too shy, traumatized or reticent to say anything about their experience. It is possible then that important perspectives are missing. Likewise, the time pressures within clinics meant I encountered difficulties in interviewing the medical staff; they simply had little time to indulge me. This is a subject worth pursuing in the future. This study is also Bangkok-based; although I have no reason to believe that assisted reproduction clinics differ greatly across Thailand, it does mean that the majority of my informants are Central Thai urban elites, rather than people from other regions. Finally, of course, are all the attendant difficulties of interpretation and translation across languages and cultures. No doubt despite my best efforts and the erstwhile assistance of my friend and colleague Som who accompanied me to all interviews, there are subtleties missed, questions poorly asked and answers misunderstood.

Ethical clearance to conduct the project was received from the University of Melbourne Human Research Ethics Committee (HREC 060504X.2), the Faculty of Medicine, Mahidol University (016/2550) and clearances obtained through all participating hospitals and clinics and the National Research Council of Thailand (No. 0002.3/2069).

8. Appadurai's (1996: 31) '-scapes' include: ethnoscapes, referring to the landscape of mobile people such as migrants and tourists; technoscapes, consisting of the global configuration of technology that moves rapidly across various boundaries; finanscapes, or the 'disposition of global capital'; mediascapes, referring to the distribution of information electronically and the images of the world and lives created by it; and ideascapes that 'frequently have to do with the ideologies of the state and the counter-ideologies of other social movements concerned with capturing state power.

Chapter 1

The Birth of IVF in Thailand

> Everything went well until about 36–37 weeks of pregnancy; I received a call from the mother around 10–11 PM telling me that she had amniotic fluid. She was in Korat at the time so I was very nervous and told them to rush to Bangkok. I got everything ready for the operation because I did not want to wait until it was too late. I did not get any sleep from 10–11 PM that night until dawn. I could not get to sleep so I came here to prepare everything. There were about five or six doctors, anaesthesiologists and nurses ready so we could get started as soon as she arrived. She did not turn up until almost midday. I was … [so worried] … but she told me that she did not see any point of coming so soon. In the operating room, nurses and everyone were surprised that there were so many doctors, nurses, anaesthesiologists and paediatricians for this case. People were so interested but I told them that I would explain later. –Professor Pramuan Virutamasen, the 'Father of IVF' in Thailand

It is over twenty-five years since the arrival of Thailand's first IVF baby, 'Mung Ming', from Chulalongkorn Hospital in 1987. The pregnancy was announced with nationalistic pride as a scientific triumph. Thai success with IVF came less than a decade after the birth of Louise Brown in 1978 in Britain. The second IVF birth came in Australia in 1980 and the third in the United States in 1982. When Thailand's first IVF-conceived child was finally safely delivered at thirty-seven weeks gestation on 15 August, he was declared 'completely healthy' and the parents 'very happy' after trying to have a baby for five years. Professor Pramuan was asked to name the boy and to be the 'god father' (บิดาอุปถัมภ์). He was named Pawornwit

Srisaburi (ปวรวิทย์ ศรีสหบุรี). As Professor Pramuan explained: 'His name is Pawornwit. The letter 'P' was from the first character of my name and the letter 'w' was from the first character of the first name of another doctor who was helping me' (Dr Wisut Boonkasemsanti). Four days after the birth, the proud parents displayed their baby boy to the awaiting press.

This chapter charts the history of IVF in Thailand by describing various key moments in the public lives of these technologies. At one level, it is a history dominated by scientific 'firsts', celebrity cases and debates over ethical dilemmas posed by the new technologies. These helped define infertility as a treatable 'disease' and created new categories of 'patients' and a proliferation of new meanings attached to infertility, family, reproduction and technology (De Rosa et al. 2003). But it is also a history that includes events that posed serious challenges to the public perception of IVF doctors as brilliant and benevolent. Most of all, what this chapter demonstrates is the gradual 'naturalization' (Lock and Kaufert 1998: 19) of these technologies into the reproductive repertoire of Thai couples. This chapter draws upon extensive media material from both Thai and English language newspapers, books and Internet sources. It also draws upon an in-depth interview with Professor Pramuan Virutamasen, a leading figure in the history of IVF in Thailand, as well as informal discussions with other reproductive specialists. No attempt has been made to conceal identities in this chapter as all are already reported in the public domain.

Population Governance in Thailand

To understand the history of assisted reproduction in Thailand it is necessary to briefly lay out the broader dimensions of the biopolitics shaping reproduction in Thai society. One fundamental 'Asian value' evoked by the state is that of 'the family'. The management of population size, growth and composition is a powerful domain of governance (Foucault 1984) and in Thailand there is a long history of interventions by the state into the reproductive lives of citizens – the form of the family, encouraging or regulating population and safe sexual behaviour. An effect of these interventions is to stratify reproduction (Ginsburg and Rapp 1991) – produce political and economic constraints which structure reproductive decisions.

The form of the family has always been a concern of the governments of Siam/Thailand. Sakdina[1] laws dating back to the fifteenth century in Thailand defined social categories of people and the rights they were entitled to in terms of land and people and maintained social distinctions by policing the boundaries of female sexuality and marriage. As Tamara Loos (1999) documents, from the late 1700s to the late 1800s the Three Seals Law was the most important legal text which contained a series of laws governing sexuality, marriage and the social recognition of children. It also included direct references to reproductive issues. Following the administrative reforms of King Chulalongkorn's reign, the legal system in Thailand underwent a series of reforms from the 1890s to 1930s resulting in the modern penal and civil code, including family laws.

The institution of the family became an especially important site for notions of Thainess and nation building in Siam under the reign of King Vajiravudh (Rama VI, r. 1910–1925) who wrote a series of essays on family and sexuality, linking the form of the family with notions of civilization, progress and nation building (Loos 1999: 238). The legal reforms of his reign narrowly defined the family in terms of a stable long-term union between a man and his legitimate wife or wives. New laws regulated sexuality by defining any sex outside of publicly recognized unions as immoral. Reforms instituted in the 'Modern Family Law' described by Loos included a range of requirements shaping the form of the family, the replacement of polygyny with monogamy as the legal form of marriage and the introduction of medical notions of impotency, sterility and puberty into laws under the category of 'defective sexual organs' as grounds for divorce (Loos 1999: 251). Such laws denote increasing involvement of the state in the form of families and sexual and reproductive relations.

Following the Second World War, the Thai government under Prime Minister Phibulsongkram pursued an agenda of pronatalist nationalism and modernization. On 9 March 1956 the premier 'called on the men and women of Thailand to build up the country's population to 40 million' (*Bangkok Post*, 10). Unmarried people were viewed as 'unproductive consumers'. During his rule, a deliberate nation-building strategy to develop Thainess was imposed. The twelve cultural mandates (*rathniyom*) issued between 1939 and 1942 targeted the behaviour and comportment of women, including within marriage. Motherhood was promoted as the patriotic duty of women as 'flowers of the nation' celebrated through a National Mother's Day (Van Esterik 2000). Policies promoted large families especially among the educated classes through schemes giving higher wages to government employees with large families (*Bangkok Post*, 27 April

1957). The current abortion law came into effect at this time, which only permitted abortion in cases where it endangered a woman's health (Whittaker 2004). The pronatalist government position continued through the subsequent Sarit military regime.

This stance changed in the late 1960s with the emergence of a new discourse in the West which viewed rapid population growth as a global 'population problem' of great urgency. The advent of new 'modern' forms of contraceptives was seen to provide a means of controlling population growth. In 1968 the prime minister signed the United Nations' World Leaders Declaration on Population and in that same year the cabinet permitted family health services to be extended to married women with children throughout the Kingdom, a move publicly endorsed by the king of Thailand. In March 1970 the Thai cabinet had declared the first family planning policy in Thailand linking reproductive decision making directly with the economic and social progress of the state, thereby reversing its previous pronatalist position: 'The government has the policy to support voluntary family planning in order to resolve various problems concerned with the very high rate of population growth which constitutes an important obstacle to the economic and social development of the nation' (quoted in Krannich and Krannich 1980: 18). A National Family Planning Program was incorporated into the Third National Economic and Social Development Plan (1972–1976) in which family planning was promoted not only as a means to improve the quality of life and health of Thai citizens, but for strategic economic and political objectives given the then communist insurgency in the northeast of Thailand. A vigorous program supporting family planning and access to contraceptives followed. So successful has the Thai family planning program been that it produced what has been termed by demographers a 'Demographic Revolution' which dropped the Thai fertility rate from 7.63 births per woman in 1969 to 3.82 births per women by 1984 (Knodel, Chamratrithirong and Debavalya 1987). Since then the fertility rate further dropped to 1.6 by 2007 (Mahidol Population Gazette 2007). Within such a context little attention or state support was given to the treatment of infertility, and infertile couples had few options other than adoption.

Thai IVF

An article was published in a Thai newspaper in 1978 announcing the birth of the world's first baby through IVF, Louise Brown. The article suggested that IVF was possibly unethical from a medical perspective and described a range of religious perspectives regarding the procedure. It was clearly based upon an international article as it included no local Thai Buddhist commentary.[2] The fanfare over the first test tube baby seemed another Western experiment removed from Thailand. Yet by this time Professor Pramuan Virutamasen had already begun to experiment with the collection of mouse oocytes and IVF in laboratory mice following his return from the University of Pennsylvania in 1972 (pers. comm., 2007). Professor CR Bannister from Cambridge University came to visit Thailand for six months at this time and demonstrated how to modify some basic equipment and perform in vitro culture. However, he encountered difficulties in obtaining the highly purified water required and the specific mouse species needed in Thailand and this delayed his progress. Finally, Professor Pramuan sourced water distilled from a copper tank at the Department of Physics at Chulalongkorn University, at the time not realizing that elements of copper distillate are important components of culture media. By the mid-1980s the team at Chulalongkorn was already fertilizing mouse eggs and growing their embryos. Once permission to begin work on humans was granted, the next difficulty was obtaining human oocytes, because at that time they did not have drugs such as gonadotrophin for ovarian stimulation. A young woman admitted for surgery for carcinoma donated her oocytes for the research. Professor Pramuan explained his excitement at the first success with embryos:

> I was participating in the university's anniversary at Chula on 26 March.... I came back to see that the fertilization had developed about two to three stages so far! I got other people to have a look as well.... I was so happy and proud that I succeeded. Then, I grew the second and the third ones using the same principles and that got me to think what I needed to do about transferring. The next thing is about ethic[al] issues. So many people objected and asked me what I would do with the fertilized eggs. I was confused and did not know what to do and who to transfer the eggs to. I kept growing the eggs, then, they were hatching and died. I got worried so I went to see my Abbot and asked him if this was a sin. He explained a lot of things but did not answer [my question]. I came back and continued with the work because there were so many people with infertility problems. I made the transfer to the first person. I was very happy and did not want to believe that she got pregnant, I checked her beta SCG and it got to about one to two hundred something. Later on about twelve to fourteen weeks, she had an ectopic pregnancy. It was so sad. I was so disappointed and checked back to the history of ... Patrick Setto and

> R. G. Edward in England [doctors involved with the world's first IVF baby]; they experienced the ectopic pregnancy on the first person and succeeded on the second one as well. It was exactly the same scenario. We succeeded on the second one and gave birth to the baby on 15 August 1987 ... our first [test tube] baby ... he is [now] studying third year in engineering, international programme. Then came the second one. At the time, it was quite difficult to get each baby each year. The second one is [now] studying first year medical sciences at Rama [University]. Since then, the procedures got developed very quickly.

In this narrative, Professor Pramuan describes not only his intense curiosity, scientific drive and excitement, but also the moment of realization that he now faced the ethical dilemma of growing human embryos. Although seeking advice from a member of the Buddhist clergy, none was offered and so he continued, finally transferring embryos and achieving pregnancies. The successful birth of the first IVF baby quickly legitimated his experimentation.

What is missing from his narrative is the names of his collaborators, in particular Dr Wisut Boonkasemsanti, the 'other doctor' he refers to in Pawornwit's name. In March 1992 Professor Pramuan and Professor Wisut were announced as medical award winners for their work on IVF.[3] At no time during our interview was Dr Wisut mentioned. The reason for his removal from the triumphant narrative of IVF success will be described later in this chapter.

Finally, what is apparent in this account is that the use of personal pronouns throughout clearly denotes a sense of ownership on the part of the doctor. Mung Ming was 'our first baby'. This sense of primary responsibility is maintained in the clinics where doctors frequently speak of 'their babies' and 'creating life'. Indeed, Professor Pramuan and the clinic staff maintain an interest in the lives of babies born through their assistance. When I asked about Mung Ming, he commented: 'He told me that he did not feel any inferiority. He has no problem telling everyone how he was born when he is asked. He understands that it's normal; does not think that he is a hero or anything. As far as I know, his parents told him everything from the beginning.'

Unlike the development of IVF in India where the technologies and personnel quickly transferred to the private sector (Lloyd 1996), in Thailand the major advances in reproductive technologies have been made in the public sector at major university hospitals and they retain prestige as leading centres for treatment and research. Professor Pramuan continued his work at Chulalongkorn University and remains involved in IVF at its clinic.

Movie-Star Doctors

The birth of Thailand's first IVF baby was greeted with acclaim and curiosity by the Thai public. As Dr Pramuan described it: 'Press came in as if we were movie stars.' His name continues to be synonymous with IVF and he is still the main expert approached by the press to comment on any development in assisted reproductive technology (ART). Thai press coverage of Mung Ming's birth lauded the doctors as scientific experts and presented them as primary to the process, relegating the parents to the periphery (Stanworth 1987). The doctors involved were described as 'proficient, excellent, world-class'. Unlike the religious debates that occurred with the birth of the world's first IVF baby in Britain, within Thailand little religious controversy ensued and on the whole there was nothing but positive coverage about the birth.

As Aditya Bharadwaj (2002) suggested for India's first test tube baby, there is a tendency for the babies created through such processes to be viewed as scientific trophies. Likewise, in Thailand the birth of Mung Ming was heralded as evidence of Thailand's scientific excellence and modernity. The head of the Obstetrics and Gynaecology Department, Chulalongkorn Hospital, Dr Nikon Dusitsin, declared that although other countries like Singapore and Taiwan had succeeded earlier, these countries had brought in foreign experts to conduct their IVF experiments; the effort in Thailand had been conducted only by Thais.[4] The patriotic nature of scientific endeavour was further underscored by a statement attributed to Professor Pramuan in a report in *Matichon* newspaper where he was quoted as stating that 'the reason for doing this experiment is to participate in the King's sixtieth birthday celebration and also because there are around forty infertile couples contacting him for treatment each week'.[5]

From early on, then, assisted reproduction was positioned as a positive symbol of Thai expertise and with Thainess and nationhood itself through the evocation of the Thai King (himself associated with engineering and scientific ventures).

A year after Mung Ming's birth, Thailand's second IVF baby, a girl nicknamed 'Oil', was born. Her birth was greeted with the headline, 'Chula Doctors Have Done it Again: The Second test tube baby.'[6] She was born full term, her parents requesting that she be delivered between 10 AM and 12 PM, an auspicious time determined by astrologists to ensure she would be a healthy, obedient and lucky baby.

Rapid Expansion of New Technological Possibilities

More so than in other scientific fields, each new technological development in assisted reproductive medicine in Thailand has attracted media attention reporting enthusiastically on 'celebrity' doctors and 'miraculous' births. This media interest in assisted reproduction gradually introduced a new vocabulary into Thai society. Initially the terms used in Thai for assisted reproductive techniques were confusing. In early reports the term phasom tiam ผสมเทียม (literally, 'artificial mixing') was used to describe birth artificial insemination and IVF. Gradually the term *dek lord kaew* เด็กหลอดแก้ว ('glass-tube baby') emerged to differentiate IVF from other techniques. But the term 'glass-tube baby' itself resulted in misunderstanding. According to a report in *Thai Rath* during a presentation on the first IVF birth,[7] some people wanted to see how big the test tube was that the baby was grown in. Eventually, as the novelty of IVF techniques wore off, English scientific acronyms came to be used in Thai to name the various techniques. Reports in the newspapers helped educate the public about the technologies. They more or less accurately explained the differences between artificial insemination, IVF, GIFT, ZIFT, the use of frozen sperm and frozen embryos and tried to improve the public understanding of the technologies. For instance, on 12 March 1992 *Matichon* reported on the development of hormones to stimulate the production of the lining of the uterus for implantation of the embryo. The article explained that 'the rumour that men can get pregnant is not true. Those who can get pregnant are those who have a uterus. Chula doctors can create artificial lining of the uterus, not an artificial uterus.'[8]

On 22 March 1984 Chulalongkorn Hospital established Thailand's first sperm bank. Although artificial insemination treatments using fresh sperm were available, it was the first time that frozen sperm donations could be stored for use at a later date. In particular, it provided the possibility for men with low sperm counts to gradually build up a store of sperm to be used, hence avoiding the need to use sperm from anonymous donors. In addition, the bank reportedly stored sperm donated from 'intelligent' medical students for use in cases when men had no sperm. It was reported that the service was also available for single women.[9] By 1987 it was reported that demand for the services of the bank was greater than the supply of semen available.[10] By 4 March 2001 *Thai Rath* was reporting that 'hi-society people were rushing to keep their sperm at the sperm bank'. It continued: 'Male politicians, well-known men and hi-society men are afraid of not having descendants, rushing to use services of the sperm bank at Chulalongkorn University. As a result, there is too much sperm kept there now.'[11]

The first baby born through gamete intrafallopian transfer (GIFT) was delivered in 1987 by Dr Jongjet Aojanepong at the Police Hospital; he now runs the famous private Jetanin clinic. Once again the birth was announced with a surge of nationalistic pride: 'Thai doctors succeed again.'[14] One newspaper initially reported this achievement as Thailand's first 'real IVF baby', confusing the GIFT techniques with IVF.[15] Around this time assisted reproduction entered popular culture in the form of a television soap opera, '*Umbun*', with a convoluted plot about an adopted daughter; *umbun* entered Thai vocabulary as the new term for surrogacy (see chapter 9). One newspaper report suggested that this soap opera, news stories about the test tube twins and the demand for the sperm bank had an impact upon the feelings of Thailand's orphans. It suggested that the advent of these technologies make it less likely for orphans to find adoptive parents, and as a consequence 'some of the orphans of today are a time bomb of the future', predicting that this would result in social problems (*Thairath*, 9 November 1990). The first baby born from a frozen embryo on 17 April 1991 at Chulalongkorn Hospital was reported in *Matichon* with the predictable pun: 'Thai doctors are cool again.'[16]

Although in the earliest days each IVF birth was reported, as IVF became more commonplace births of IVF babies tended to only be reported when they involved some extraordinary aspect, such as high-order multiple births. The first set of girl triplets was reported in September 1990 from Chulalongkorn Hospital to a business couple.[17] They were the eleventh IVF babies in the country and, at that time, twenty-one other couples were expecting, two of which were carrying twins. Bumrungrad Hospital reported their first case of quadruplets (their second IVF case) to a 35-year-old woman on 2 April 1992.[18] On 10 March 2005 quintuplets were born to a 'lucky' couple in Hat Yai. The quintuplets were born prematurely at thirty-one weeks, and each weighed less than two kilograms at birth. Donations of milk and money were called for and Hat Yai Hospital reported that a large number of couples contacted the hospital following their birth to enquire about IVF treatment.[19]

Although rare nowadays due to a change in clinical practices in IVF whereby fewer embryos are transferred, multiple births are still viewed positively in Thailand. Press reports of multiple births rarely spoke of the medical risks involved to mothers and children, but rather presented these instances as evidence of the bounty and merit associated with IVF.

Further technological advances in assisted reproduction continued to merit media interest. Intracytoplasmic sperm injection (ICSI) was introduced into Thailand in 1991. The injection of sperm into the cytoplasm of the ovum directly allowed men with low sperm counts or problematic sperm to father a biological child and no longer rely on donor sperm. With this technology a new group of patients was defined: that of infertile men. The director of IVF Sydney at the time visited Vichaiyut Hospital to speak about the technique and it became available at the hospital the next year (*Thairath*, 8 November 1991). The technique of using hormonal injections to assist women to develop an appropriate lining in their uteri to facilitate implantation was introduced in 1992, announced in one newspaper with the headline, 'The red light (menstruation) is off but (women) can still have a baby. Thai doctors really can do it.'[20] This report carried a warning that doctors should not encourage women who are menopausal to have a baby. The development of this technology extended the potential period of a woman's fertility and defined older women as potential patients and mothers.

Although initially confined to Bangkok, IVF technologies quickly spread throughout Thailand. In 1996 doctors outside of Bangkok (in Nakorn Pathom and in Samut Prakan) announced their first successful IVF births.[21] By the tenth anniversary of Mung Ming's birth, assisted reproductive technologies were available across the country. A tenth-anniversary reunion party marking the success of IVF was held on the fiftieth anniversary of the Faculty of Medicine at Chulalongkorn University on 25 April 1997.[22] By that time there had been 236 babies born through IVF at Chulalongkorn Hospital and a 10-metre cloth of hand-written notes of thanks was presented to staff.

A by-product of the rapid expansion of assisted reproductive technologies was the creation of a new discourse of infertility in Thailand (De Rosa et al. 2003). With the advent of each new technological intervention, new categories of 'patients', such as infertile men, older women or HIV positive men, were created and infertility itself became a 'disease' to be treated in the realm of biomedicine. The media placed infertility in public view in Thailand, representing the infertile as patients for whom technology could offer solutions, and reinforcing biology as the basis for parental ties.

Celebrity Pregnancies

Across its history, assisted reproductive technologies have also spawned their share of bizarre and sensational headlines and displays of grand or mischievous misunderstanding. Famous movie and pop stars occasionally appear in the news apparently seeking to undergo IVF to have babies with their lesbian partners or through surrogates in what appear to be either fabulous or fatuous publicity campaigns. There is no clear evidence when the first IVF surrogacy began in Thailand. It is believed to have first been undertaken at Chulalongkorn Hospital in 1991.[23] The issue of surrogacy was publicized in 1988 through the case of the actress and daughter-in-law of the then minister for foreign affairs, Mayura (มยุรา). In an article featuring a picture of her in skimpy gym clothes touching her toes, it was reported in September 1988 that she had asked her sister to be a surrogate for a child using her eggs and her husband's sperm and had already consulted doctors in the United States in Boston, MA. Now that Thai doctors had successfully birthed an IVF baby she was considering doing this in Thailand.[24] This article was followed with a short piece outlining the legal precedents such a case would set.[25] In a follow-up article to the case, Mayura denied she had paid her sister to be a surrogate mother, rather that it was something she had considered in the past when newly wedded but had since given up. She claimed that the story was simply an effort to promote her latest movie. She now felt very discouraged as a result of the negative criticism that she and her sister had received.[26]

In the late 1980s and early 90s, several television celebrities revealed their use of these technologies. Such cases served to familiarize IVF to the Thai public, but also confirmed their status as technologies for the wealthy privileged elite. These stories also reinforced a perception that infertility was a problem for the elite due to their work stress.

At times public representations of these technologies have verged on the bizarre. The challenges that these technologies pose for gender relations and notions of 'natural' reproduction is epitomized with musings over whether men can have babies. For instance in May 2000, following the successfully delivery of a Thai baby conceived naturally who developed outside the womb in an ectopic pregnancy, a series of newspaper articles reported that in principle it was now possible for men to carry pregnancies with IVF. With playful journalistic logic, prominent Thai transgender celebrities were interviewed about the possibility. One transgender personality was famous for appearing in a movie about a famous *kathoei* volleyball team *Satri lek*, 'Iron Women', who won the National Volleyball championships. She stated she would not be afraid if selected for this experiment. However, she noted that it might not be acceptable in Thai society because the baby would be born unnaturally.[27] 'Sunny', a former singer in the popular band U4, famous for announcing she would spend the rest of her life as a woman, was also interviewed and disagreed with the idea of men being pregnant.[28]

Such celebrity stories presented yet another image of the infertile as acquisitive consumers satisfying their frivolous desires through whatever means (De Rosa et al. 2003). Celebrity cases reinforced an association between assisted reproduction, the wealthy and socially deviant. They also served to introduce new forms of family and relationships into Thai imaginaries.

Murder

The story of the birth of IVF is not simply one of scientific triumph and surreal possibilities, but a history that has its own tragedies and controversies. The most tragic incident in the history of these technologies in Thailand involves the case of Dr Wisut Boonkasemsanti, one of the Chulalongkorn doctors involved in the early development of IVF and Thailand's first test tube baby. As noted earlier, part of his name was combined with that of Dr Pramuan to form the name of Thailand's first test tube baby.

On 10 November 2003 the Southern Bangkok Criminal Court sentenced Dr Wisut to death for the murder of his wife, Dr Phassaporn Boonkasemsanti, head obstetrician at the State Railway Hospital. In 1999 the couple had separated and Wisut had filed for divorce; however, Phassapon did not agree and there were said to be arguments over assets and allegations of previous violence. On 20 February 2001 Wisut asked his wife to meet him at a restaurant and following this she was not seen again. The court found that after the meal, Wisut checked into the staff hostel at Chulalongkorn University and there killed and systematically dismembered her body. He left to pick up his children from school, dropped them at her house and then visited a store to buy large black plastic bags, large paper rolls and solid deodorants. Parts of her flesh were later found in the room's septic tanks and her blood was found in the room. He had hired a woman to type letters from his wife asking for leave to go on a meditation retreat at Chantaburi for several days and other letters to her children. Her forged signature was on the letters which were sent from Nonthaburi. On 21 February Dr Wisut checked into a room at the Sofitel Hotel and on 26 March police retrieved human remains from the septic system of the Sofitel as well. Dr Wisut later filed complaints that his wife had disappeared. On 23 March 2001 Dr Wisut was charged with illegal detention and was later charged with premeditated murder. Later, the original prosecution at Southern Bangkok Criminal Court dropped charges against Dr Wisut and he was released.

However, on 5 June 2001 Dr Phassaporn's father filed a private suit against Dr Wisut for premeditated murder which was accepted by the Attorney General's Office in September 2002. In October 2002 charges were again brought against Dr Wisut in the Southern Bangkok Criminal Court and in November he was found guilty and sentenced to death. He has maintained his innocence throughout the trial. On 3 July 2005 his appeal was rejected and Bangkok's Appeal Court upheld the death sentence. He did not receive a royal pardon in June 2006 in commemoration of the sixtieth anniversary of the king's reign as his case was under appeal. On 25 July 2007 the Supreme Court upheld the death sentence against him (*Bangkok Post*, 26 July 2007). On 12 December 2007 the *Bangkok Post* announced that his sentence had been reduced to life imprisonment as part of a royal pardon given by His Majesty the King to mark his eightieth birthday.

Up until this case, IVF doctors were only ever associated with life-affirming, positive and meritorious characteristics. This case served to discredit the image of the benevolent doctor, replacing it with the grisly voyeurism of detailed descriptions of the murder and dismemberment of the body. As noted earlier, when I interviewed Professor Pramuan in 2007, Dr Wisut's name was not mentioned once in his recounting the history of IVF in Thailand.

The reaction among many former patients of Dr Wisut was one of disbelief. A number of his patients, including the parents of the first test tube baby, came out in his public defence stating in the media that he was a good man not capable of such a thing. The inability of some of his patients to believe the charges against him illustrates the power of the relationship created between infertility patients and their doctors, as shown in the following comments posted anonymously to the Thai message board *mthai*:[29]

> We all have to take responsibilities of our own actions ... the doctor is still in many of his student's and patients hearts. May the doctor be at peace. (Comment 11)

> I feel sorry for him. His punishment should get reduced because he has done so many good things in his life. He could be a prison doctor. (Comment 43)

> Why execution? A good person like him should live. At least, he is a good father to his children. I am on your side. (Comment 178, signed *rakmormak*, 'love the doctor a lot')

In 2003 another legal case prominent in the press involved the actions of a 73-year-old Bangkok doctor. Dr Narathorn Thammabutr confessed to undertaking GIFT treatment on women and convincing them they were pregnant while continuing to treat them with a range of injections and medicines at a high cost.[30] Three patients lodged a case against him. One patient had submitted herself to seventy-six injections and spent over 110,000 baht (approximately US $30,000). The Thai Medical Council revealed that Dr Thammabutr was in fact trained as a microbiologist and had been retired for a number of years, though all they had the power to do if he was found guilty was to withdraw his registration for two years. The doctor closed his clinic and pleaded guilty.

Such cases disrupted the public narrative of infertility doctors as wise and benevolent. Given that there were no regulations governing assisted reproduction in Thailand during this time, these doctors held ethical responsibility for the application of the technologies. Negative publicity regarding a few doctors undermined the trust placed in their profession.

Ethical Issues

Assisted reproductive technologies pose new ethical issues for Thais to consider. For the most part, in contrast to the issue of abortion, there has been very limited public debate in the media about the ethics of assisted reproductive technologies. It was not until January 1998 (eleven years after Mung Ming's birth) that an initial Medical Council Order was published in the Royal Gazette requiring all clinics undertaking IVF to provide counselling to patients to prepare them for possible problems and requiring clinics to appoint an ethical committee to decide on treatments and medications.

The few pronouncements from leading monks on the ethics of assisted reproduction have been generally supportive of these technologies as meritorious and life affirming allowing an opportunity for the rebirth of a soul that otherwise might not have taken place.

Within the media, there has been limited debate over issues such as the use of these technologies for gay and lesbian couples and single women, the availability of commercial surrogacy and the trade in ova, and no discussion of clinical practices such as the disposal of embryos or use in research, foetal reduction or social sex selection. For the most part, the Thai public seems generally unaware of the range of practices available within Thailand and until recently has not questioned the self-regulation of clinical practice by clinics' ethics committees.

At the time of Mung Ming's birth, Major General Chamlong Srimuang, then Bangkok governor, was asked about the Buddhist ethical position with regards to IVF. As I described in my previous work on abortion (Whittaker 2004), Chamlong was a prominent member of the Santi Asoke Buddhist sect which was highly active in the campaigns throughout the 1980s against abortion-law reform. He was noted for positioning himself as a moral crusader. His response largely reflected a common heroic representation of assisted reproduction as life giving versus abortion as life destroying: 'IVF treatment is not against Buddhist principles as we don't kill, steal or sleep with married women/men. As long as they don't mix whatever in the tube (which is like sleeping with married women or men) and as long as they stick with one husband, one wife, they don't do anything wrong. However, abortion is clearly against Buddhist principles as it is killing' (*Matichon,* 31 May 1987).

His suggestion failed to provoke any further discussion. His response reflects a limited understanding of the various techniques used at that time in Thailand, such as the use of donor gametes, equating the mixing of gametes as equivalent to having sexual intercourse with married men or women. It also shows how issues such as embryo wastage, embryo donation and fetal reduction have been avoided in public discourse on IVF in Thailand.

The issue of paternity continues to carry unease in Thailand in the use of IVF technologies. In particular, the desire for single women or lesbian couples to produce a baby through the use of intrauterine insemination (IUI) or IVF attracts criticism from doctors and the public whenever it arises in the media. Within the public discourse, only heterosexually married couples are considered appropriate candidates to become mothers. In October 2000 the case of Philaiphan Bunlon, nicknamed 'Mam', a successful businesswoman and managing director of a media company and her partner, former Thai actress Arunothai Jittrikhan or 'Nong', caused public condemnation when they announced their intention to have an heir by using her egg and the sperm of a foreign donor to create a blastocyst to be carried in the womb of her partner. Thai doctors reputedly refused to assist and hence she stated she would pursue treatment overseas. A fertility specialist, Dr Thongthit Thongyai, gave a patronizing analysis of the reasons why single women are interested in IVF, which not only ignored the issues of social infertility or homosexuality but highlights a common construction of children as companions and marriage to Thai men as problematic. He suggested:

> We want them (single women) to think long-term, not only think that they need to have a friend, or a doll to be their company. When these children were born, they will be asked who their father is. [Single women desire children] ... because they are afraid of being lonely. They don't know for whom they have to live their life or to whom they will give their inheritance. Importantly, most single ladies are afraid of a rocky married life, divorce, and an unfaithful husband and don't want to be upset when marriage ends. In addition, they are confident that they can look after themselves and their family and they don't have to rely on men.[31]

'Not like the US': Debating Limits

The growth of assisted reproductive technologies in Thailand prompted a range of ethical dilemmas, particularly as techniques involving donor ova and surrogacy became more common. In October 2001 the Medical Association of Thailand hosted a debate entitled, 'What society thinks about the egg, sperm and embryo trade?' Discussions such as these marked recognition of the need for further regulation of the use of assisted reproductive technologies and contributed to the development of a draft bill (discussed below). The demand for assisted reproductive technologies had spawned a lucrative market in Thailand and there was recognition that the lack of legislation might need to be addressed. At this meeting it was noted that there was a growing ambiguity between altruistic donation of eggs, sperm and embryos and commercial practice. The president of medical ethics noted that a trade existed in Thailand and is attracting foreigners seeking these services.[32] He noted that 'this kind of trade is like abortion which is available every day and everywhere although it's illegal' and noted at least five hospitals that were involved. 'If this business keeps expanding, one day we will be like the US where they trade openly.'[33] All discussants suggested that such trade should be illegal. Draft legislation was discussed using the concept of *borijak,* a donation that brings with it merit to the giver.

The comment warning that Thailand should not become 'like the US' reveals another theme that frequently emerges in discussion of assisted reproductive technologies in Thailand. The image of the West as the source of moral corruption of Thai values has a long history in Thailand, and such comments draw upon well-rehearsed imagery. It was a common theme in debates of abortion-law reform (Whittaker 2004). It is not surprising that on another biopolitical topic concerning the status of embryos and the nature of the family, Thai Buddhist values were once again contrasted with those of the West. It emerged again in reports of the possibility of genetically modified babies following the announcement in the United States that babies had been born following a technique where cytoplasm from a donor egg was injected into the mother's egg. This resulted in the transfer of some genetic material from the donor egg into the mother's egg, so that babies could develop with genetic material from three people. The Thai government was urged to legislate to curb the use of such techniques, with one commentator in *BizWeek*[34] comparing the genetic modification of children to Nazism.[35] Assisted reproduction had thus moved from a discourse of wondrous science and benevolent doctors to Frankensteinian scenarios.

The Drafting of Assisted Reproductive Technologies Legislation in Thailand

Until 2014 the use of assisted reproductive technologies in Thailand was very loosely regulated. The need for legislation to regulate assisted reproductive practice was suggested as early as 1987. A seminar at Chulalongkorn Hospital pointed to the need for legal protection of the rights of children born through these procedures and to prevent commercial surrogacy.[36] Although the Thai Medical Council introduced professional guidelines in 1997 and 2001 for assisted reproductive technologies, including surrogacy, these lacked legal force.

The drafting of new legislation took many years. In 1997 the *Bangkok Post* announced that new legislation to protect the rights of children born through artificial insemination and other methods would be introduced by the end of the year following support from the National Youth Bureau.[37] By 2000 a Thai Medical Council public seminar of representatives from the Department of Religious Affairs, Law Council, Nursing Council and various academics discussed the need for legislation to avoid a 'chaotic and confused society', as assisted reproductive technologies and surrogacy had caused 'social problems'.[38] This seminar was in response to reports that several legal cases had arisen involving children born through assisted reproductive technologies challenging Thai legal definitions of family, kinship and inheritance.[39]

Once again in 2001 newspapers reported plans for legislation regulating assisted reproduction and surrogacy.[40] By 2004 further reports of progress on the draft appeared in the newspaper following a seminar on surrogacy law held by the Ministry of Social Development and Human Security. A series of public hearings regarding the proposed legislation were held throughout 2005 around the country and female members of parliament were said to be in support of the draft bill.[41] In 2006 it was announced that the draft legislation was prepared and would focus firstly on the child's interests, morality, culture and values in Thai society as priorities and finally consider the needs and rights of biological parents, surrogate mothers, agents and doctors who provide treatment without impeding any future technological advancement.[42] One participant in the drafting of the legislation stated: 'Legislation can't keep up with ARTs, creating a problem whether the baby is a legal baby and will have legal rights such as using a surname, right to get inheritance. When parents agree to use these technologies, they have to take/accept this child for the rest of their lives without having feelings that this child is not theirs. If they don't, this may make the child have no faith in life and become the second class citizen in society.'

When details of the new draft legislation were released in 2008, public discussion ensued. The proposed surrogacy laws were especially scrutinized. The Women's Health Advocacy Foundation stated that 'the aim of the legislation is meant to look after surrogate mothers and children but in fact, not only does it fail to do so but also pushes the burden to the surrogate mothers'.[43] The draft bill was approved by the Thai cabinet as part of bill 167/2553, the Assisted Reproductive Technologies Bill, in May 2010 but political instability further delayed its progress. It was not until 2014 that a series of controversies stimulated action.

Rotten Trade

A series of events involving the growth of an international trade in reproductive services in Thailand finally prompted the introduction of legislation. Assisted reproduction has become increasingly globalized as people travel to undertake treatment across borders. With its relative lack of regulation on assisted reproduction, Thailand became popular as a destination for couples seeking the availability of surrogates and ova donors.[44] Although Thailand is not alone in this market, it became a hub for such travel in the region, a topic I describe elsewhere (Whittaker 2008, 2009, 2012). The difficulties of regulating an increasingly global reproductive trade became evident to the Thai public in a series of highly publicized events that revealed a 'rotten trade' (Bhagwati 2002)[45] in reproductive services.

The first of these occurred in January 2011 when Thai police raided a house in a suburb of Bangkok run by the Taiwanese company 'Baby 101'[46] revealing the organized trafficking of Vietnamese women for surrogacy to produce babies for Taiwanese couples. At the time of the raid, thirteen Vietnamese women were rescued, and a further two women were identified, one at a hospital after just having given birth. The women were held in two houses in Bangkok during their surrogacy and had their passports confiscated and movement restricted. Eleven women said they had volunteered to work as surrogates for US $5,000 per surrogacy. Four women said they had been tricked into the work. Seven of the women were pregnant, one with twins. Two of the women who were eighteen weeks pregnant sought to abort their pregnancies but were refused permission to do so.

On 22 June 2012 the Thai Primary Court found all five defendants in the case guilty as charged. One Taiwanese woman was sentenced to 5.3 years jail for human trafficking, conspiracy to detain/confine other persons and working in the Kingdom without a work permit, and a 220,000 Baht fine (US $7,040) for hiring illegal migrants. Another three Taiwanese defendants were sentenced to 5.3 years jail for human trafficking, conspiracy to detain/confine other persons and working in the Kingdom without a work permit, and a Chinese defendant was sentenced to 3 months jail for working in the Kingdom without a work permit. Three Burmese housekeepers arrested at the time were sent back to Myanmar. The Taiwanese leader of the organization has not been charged (Alliance Anti Trafic [AAT] 2012). The outcome of a Medical Council investigation into the two doctors and two hospitals involved for unethical conduct is as yet unknown.[47]

The Vietnamese women were returned to Vietnam under the auspices of various protection agencies to give birth in Vietnam. Several women continued to negotiate with the surrogacy ring to be paid for the children they birthed. After protracted negotiations and legal processes, at the end of November 2011 Ha Noi's People Committee Department of Justice signed a decision to allow eleven babies involved to be returned to their eight biological families. The Department of Immigration issued passports on 2 December and on 11 December the eleven babies arrived safely in Taiwan to their biological parents (Alliance Anti Trafic [AAT] Vietnam 2011).

Press accounts of the existence of 'baby farms' within Thailand evoked shock and reinforced calls for better regulation, particularly with regard to surrogacy. The case highlighted the lack of oversight and monitoring by clinics, the commodification of surrogacy and the vulnerability of poor women in the region to the growing trade. The trafficking of women had clear parallels with the sex trade in Thailand. The involvement of Thai doctors and hospitals, whether wittingly or unwittingly, in this scheme again unsettled confidence in the protocols and ethical standards operating in Thai clinics. Despite public outrage within the Thai press at the time, this case prompted no widespread investigation into the industry.

Other controversial cases in 2014 drew public attention to flagrant breaches of medical guidelines, potential exploitation and legal ambiguities surrounding the international assisted reproductive trade in Thailand. The first of these was a report in July 2014 on non-medical sex selection which found a number of clinics advertising sex selection services in breach of Thai Medical Council guidelines – an investigation was launched into twelve 'targeted' clinics.[48] Meanwhile, there was an ongoing highly publicised case of Israeli intending parents whose babies born through surrogacy arrangements were stranded in Thailand as the Israeli government refused to grant them citizenship.[49] In August 2014 another story broke in the media of a Japanese man, Mitsutoki Shigeta, who reportedly fathered fifteen babies to multiple surrogate mothers in Thailand and had fled the country with at least three of the babies. The clinic involved in his case, ALL-IVF was closed pending investigation.[50] At the time of writing police were still investigating this case and the doctor involved had had his case for indictment delayed four times.[51]

Baby Gammy

But of all the stories about surrogacy in Thailand in 2014, the story of Baby Gammy drew worldwide attention to the practice of international surrogacy across borders, the complex legal and ethical issues it poses, and the laxity of regulations in Thailand. In August 2014, the media ran the story of Baby Gammy, a baby boy with Down's syndrome who had been abandoned in Thailand by his Australian intended parents (and biological father) to be cared for by his gestational surrogate.[52] His twin sister had been taken back to Australia. The story broke after appeals from the surrogate, Ms Janbua Pattharamon, for support for Baby Gammy's medical expenses from international donors. She appeared in the media explaining that she had agreed to be a surrogate to pay off family debts and had refused an (illegal) abortion when it was discovered that one of the twins she was carrying had Down syndrome. She stated she had never met the intended parents and was still owed 70, 000 Baht (AUD$2,341) by the surrogacy agency. Rather than institutionalise the boy child, she offered to care for him. The intending parents took the daughter and left the country, leaving the son with the surrogate mother.[53]

In the days that followed, public disbelief and moral outrage condemned the Australian couple involved and international surrogacy in general. Editorials called for the enforcement of bans against international surrogacy.[54] Following further media investigations it was revealed that the father in the case, David Farnell is a convicted sex offender who spent time in prison for sexually abusing young girls and Australian authorities were continuing investigations into the welfare of Baby Gammy's sister. Several hundred thousand dollars was raised in funds to support Baby Gammy who became an Australian citizen in January 2015.[55]

The controversy in Australia continued when in August 2014, it was revealed in the media that another unnamed Australian man had been charged with the sexual abuse of his twin daughters conceived through surrogacy in Thailand. The couple divorced in 2008. He was the biological father of the girls. In a media interview the Thai surrogate stated she was horrified to hear of the case and open to possibly raising the girls.[56]

Reactions in Thailand: new legislation

The avalanche of horrific media reports on practices surrounding commercial surrogacy in Thailand forced the government to act. On 22 July 2014, the National Peace and Order Council (NPOC) (the military government formed following a coup d'état on 22 May 2014) announced a review of all 12 Thai IVF clinics involved in surrogacy cases believed to be possibly involved in breaches of the Thai

Medical Council guidelines and not certified by the Royal College of Obstetricians. One clinic was immediately shut down for infringing laws governing health care institutions and medical ethics.

The next act of the NPOC was to revive the Assisted Reproductive Technologies Bill number 167/2553 and move to promulgate it as law. With regard to surrogacy the new draft Assisted Reproductive Technologies Bill sets a number of conditions (these are discussed further in chapter 9) but primarily the legislation enforces a ban on commercial surrogacy or ova donation and disallows intermediaries or brokers for surrogacy arrangements.

At the time of writing, debate was continuing but the bill has been approved in principle by the current military government, and passed by the House of Representatives. It is expected to be approved by the king and promulgated sometime in 2015.[57]

Changing Representations of Reproductive Technologies

From their advent, medically assisted reproductive technologies in Thailand quickly became associated with positive imagery of science, modernity, high technology and strong maternal desire. The announcement of Thailand's first 'test tube baby' was greeted with nationalistic pride, a demonstration of the home-grown genius of Thailand's scientists and modernity. 'Infertilty' was invented as a potentially treatable medical condition, not a permanent social status, shifting from the permanent state of *khum* ('sterility') to *mi luk yak* ('difficulty having children'). Media reports have gushed over each phase in the development of these technologies, fascinated with the new imaginaries they posit for forming a family. The associations with high-tech modernity and consumerism are evident in the following quote from Dr Phoonsak Waikhwamdi, an infertility specialist, who suggests that IVF technologies have become a fashionable form of conception: 'At present, some people tend to think that natural conception is not cool; it has to be IVF, GIFT, ICSI, twins etc. They have forgotten that all of these are associated with risks for example, pre-mature delivery' (Threechana and Pimonsing 2004: 103–104).

Margaret Lock suggests that 'if the application of reproductive technologies does not coincide rather closely with widely shared societal values, they may well be judged as disruptive to the moral order, no matter how well packaged and promoted' (1998: 234). In the absence of any major misgivings from the Buddhist clergy, assisted reproductive technologies in Thailand have been represented as life affirming and supportive of the 'family'. This can be seen in comparisons between representations of assisted reproductive technologies and abortion, wherein abortion is depicted as a direct threat to Thai moral values (Whittaker 2004). From its earliest days, representations of assisted reproduction reinforced local gendered ideologies of the importance of motherhood to women as a source of female Buddhist merit and patriarchal concerns with the continuity of the patrilineage. The technologies of assisted reproduction were depicted as complementing women's desires to be mothers, a social good facilitated by benevolent male doctors. This is especially the case when upper middle class married heterosexual women use these technologies, prepared to pursue whatever means available to become mothers. Through their association with fulfilled parental desires and beautiful babies, representations of these technologies serve to reinforce rather than challenge Thai moral values.

The image of IVF doctors was tarnished by the conviction of Dr Wisut of murder. The unquestioned benevolent authority and trust of doctors came into question. Likewise, the advent of a commercial market for surrogacy and ova further complicated its representations as it runs counter to Thai values of motherhood as nurturing and sacrifice, not a commercial exchange. Once again the West was evoked as an example of the decline of moral standards. Yet as will be described later in this book in chapter 9, even surrogacy shows signs of naturalization into Thai notions of reproduction, although tension remains over its commodification. Because surrogacy dramatically confronts people with a division between biological and social parenthood it remains the most challenging to Thai moral worlds and has forced fundamental reconsideration of Thai legal definitions of motherhood. Discussions of commercialization of surrogacy in the press and the illegal trafficking of women for surrogacy highlighted a darker side to assisted reproduction and the potential exploitation of women.

More than twenty years after the birth of Mung Ming, a bill regulating the use of assisted reproductive technologies was passed by the Thai House of Representatives in 2015. At the time of writing, this legislation has still not been promulgated. It might be assumed that the lack of regulations regarding medically assisted reproductive technologies was due to a failure of legislators to keep up with technologies, and to a certain extent it is true that the rapid advances in reproductive technologies tested the speed of regulators' responses.

One might also consider what incentives the medical profession has to push for regulation in an environment where the lack of regulations has proven very profitable for them. Information about the practice of IVF particularly in private clinics has largely remained confidential and viewed as privileged information between a doctor and patient. Only when a series of controversies forced action did the NPOC act. These cases brought doctors themselves to question the moral standards of their peers.

Assisted reproductive technology has attracted the attention of the Thai press and public in ways in which few other medical advances have done. As this chapter has shown, they have become a discursive site, a 'rhetorical vehicle' (De Rosa et al. 2003) for the examination and critique of a range of social changes and modernity in Thai society: delays in childbearing due to changing roles of women, changing desires and expectations for education and careers, families within same-sex relationships, constructions of children, Buddhist ethics, medical ethics, consumerism, 'Asian family values', the very 'nature' of motherhood, even nationalism. More recent events have forced the Thai public to consider the consequences of globalisation and the potential for exploitation of Thai women's bodies in a global intimate industry. People affected by infertility and using assisted reproductive technologies bring a different range of meanings and representations to these technologies even as they negotiate the various public representations of the technology and of infertility. The varying responses of real individuals and couples and their efforts to negotiate these technologies forms the focus of the following chapters.

Notes

1. See *Thai Rath,* 19 August 1987, เด็กหลอดแก้วไทย'คลอด : สมบูรณ์ทุกประการ ผลงานแพทย์ไทย, 'Delivered Thai Test Tube Baby: Completely Healthy. The achievement of "Thai Doctors"'; and Thai Rath, 20 August 1987, แม่รายแรกเผยความรู้สึกผสมเทียม, 'First (case) Mother Reveals Her Feeling about IVF/Artificial Fertilisation.'
2. *Sakdina* translates as 'field power' or 'control over the rice field' and refers to a social system that defined each citizen in terms of the correspondence between the units of land and number of people to which that person was entitled.
3. The current criminal code and regulations regarding abortion make it illegal except in cases of a women's physical health or in cases of rape or

incest. Amendments to the abortion regulations in 2006 have relaxed these restrictions to make it possible for women to obtain legal abortions in the case of rape, foetal impairment or for mental health reasons (Royal Thai Government Gazette 2005).

4. *Thai Rath,* 28 July 1978, 'May be Medically Unethical.'
5. *Daily News,* 21 March 1992, ลูก'เทียม' งานเด่น หมอจุฬา, *'"Artificial" Baby, Outstanding Research Work, Chula Doctors.'*
6. See *Thai Rath,* 4 June 1987, หญิงไร้บุตรรุมฝากความหวังหมอเด็กหลอดแก้ว, 'Childless Women Leave their Hope (life) with Test Tube Baby Doctor'; and Ban Muang, 28 May 1987, จุฬาฯ สำเร็จ เด็กหลอดแก้ว, 'Chula Successfully Created a Test Tube Baby.'
7. *Matichon,* 28 May 1987, หมอไทยฝีมือระดับโลก ผลิตเด็กหลอดแก้วสำเร็จ, 'World-class Thai Doctors Successfully Created a Test Tube Baby.'
8. *Thai Rath,* 1 March 1989, แพทย์จุฬาฯ ทำได้อีก เด็กหลอดแก้วคนที่, '2 Chula Doctors Have Done it Again: The Second Test Tube Baby.'
9. *Thai Rath,* 4 June 1987, หญิงไร้บุตรรุมฝากความหวังหมอเด็กหลอดแก้ว, 'Childless Women Leave their Hope (Life) with Test Tube Baby Doctor.'
10. *Matichon,* 12 March 1992, เด็กหลอดแก้วแช่แข็ง, 'Frozen IVF Baby.'
11. *Thai Rath,* 23 March 1984, เชื้อน้อยฝากสะสมได้ อยากมีลูกเบิกไปทันที ขณะนี้มีหญิงท้องแล้ว, '(Men with) few sperms can store their sperms and when they would like to have a baby, they can use them right away. Five women are now pregnant.'
12. *Matichon,* 19 November 1987, 'แบงก์อสุจิ' ขายดี 'น้ำเชื้อ'ขาดแคลน, 'Outselling Sperm Bank, Short of Semen.'
13. *Thai Rath,* 4 March 2001, 'Hi-society People Rushing to Keep their Sperms at Sperm Bank.'
14. *Thai Rath,* 12 January 1990, หมอเก่ง "จุฬา-ตร." ผสมเทียมเด็กได้อีก, 'Proficient Chu la-Police (hospital) Doctors Created More (IVF/GIFT) Babies.'
15. *Naewna,* 4 July 1989, เด็กหลอดแก้วแท้สำเร็จรายแรก ฝีมือ 2 แพทย์โรงพยาบาลตำรวจ, 'Real First IVF Baby: The Work of Two Doctors at Police Hospital.'
16. *Matichon,* 6 May 1991, แพทย์ไทยเจ๋งอีก แช่แข็งได้ 3 เดือน เชื้อเด็กหลอดแก้ว, 'Thai Doctors are Cool Again. Embryo developing to be IVF baby can be frozen for 3 months.'
17. *Matichon,* 22 September 1990, ร.พ. จุฬาฯ ทำสำเร็จเด็กหลอดแก้วแฝด, '3 Chula Hospital Successfully Created IVF Triplets.'
18. *Daily News,* 2 April 1992, ผสมเทียมรายใหม่ได้แฝด, '4 New IVF Babies – Quadruplets.'
19. *Daily News,* 10 March 2005, คลอดแฝด *5 'เด็กหลอดแก้ว' :* พ่อแม่เฮงได้สมใจ, *'Khlod faed 5 "dek lord kaew", Deliver Quintuplets "Test Tube Babies": Lucky Mum and Dad getting what they Desire.'*
20. *Thairath,* 12 March 1992.
21. *Daily News,* 30 August 1996, เสนาะ ปลื้มหมอนครปฐมทำเด็กหลอดแก้วสำเร็จแล้ว, 'Proud – Nakorn Pathom Doctors Successfully Created IVF

Baby'; and Thai Rath, 9 February 1996, หมอชานเมืองเก่งผสมเทียมเด็กหลอดแก้ว เด็กคลอดแข็งแรง, 'Excellent Regional/Provincial Doctors Created an IVF Baby: The Baby was Delivered and is Healthy.'

22. *Thai Rath,* 25 April 1997, เด็กหลอดแก้วคนแรกของไทย, 'The First Test Tube Baby of Thailand.'
23. Kittiampha Kakham, 1 February 1994, *Krungthep thurakhit, 2,* อุ้มบุญให้เกิดหนทางของผู้มีลูกยาก, '*Surrogacy* Opens a Window for the Infertile.'
24. *Thai Rath,* 12 September 1988, 'Mayura Would Like to have a Baby: Asking her Sister to be a Surrogate Mother.'
25. *Thai Rath,* 12 September 1988, 'Identifying Problems (concerning the fact that) Mayura Would Like to have a Baby.'
26. *Daily News,* 21 September 1988, 'Mayura Denied that she Paid her Sister to Carry her Child'; *Daily News,* 28 September 1988, 'Nu Tuk is Discouraged about Artificial Fertilisation.'
27. *Daily News,* 3 May 2000, ฮือฮาแพทย์ไทย ยืนยัน "ผู้ชายก็ท้องได้", 'Talk of the Town: Thai Doctors Insist Male can get Pregnant.'
28. *Matichon,* 4 June 2000, ซันนี่ ยูโฟร์ ไม่เห็นด้วยผู้ชายท้อง, 'Sunny, U4 doesn't Agree that M en should get Pregnant.'
29. See http://www.mthai.com/webboard/5/117677.html, อุทธรณ์ – ฟังไม่ขึ้น ประหาร "หมอวิสุทธิ" ฆ่าเมีย (Appeal – lame, execute "Dr Wisut" [who] killed his wife). Accessed July 2006. Reactions to the case also highlighted an underlying misogynist attitude towards gender-based violence in Thailand blaming the victim and excusing his act of murder as a result of provocation by his wife:

    > Have you ever thought that it might be the doctor's wife who had done something to push him until he had to kill her. I have followed the news and it seems that his wife is not such an angel herself. (Comment 125)
    >
    > If Dr Wisut did not kill Dr Passaporn, she would kill him. Only people who know the real story know why Dr Wisut had to do such a thing. (Comment 173)
    >
    > I am so sorry for the doctor. Sometimes, a man gave everything to his wife but what he got back from her is totally opposite. ... I understand the doctor and want to tell those who curse him that even though he killed his wife but he is still better than those who murder for things, rapists, drug dealers and politicians. (Comment 183)

30. *Daily News,* 12 December 2003, 1, 14, 'Victims of Illegal GIFT Treatment Prepared to Take Legal Action. Doctors Concerned with Cancer'; *Kom Chut Leuk,* 10 December 2003, 1, 15, 'Taking Legal Action against Illegal GIFT: Verdict on February 2004'; *Kom Chut Leuk,* 13 December 2003, 1, 14, 'Argue with GIFT Victims that the Medicine Given didn't Make them Fat: They were Fat because they Took Supplements'; *Bangkok Post,* 12 December 2003, 'Fertility Doctor Accused of Raising False Hopes.'
31. *Thai Post,* 6 October 2000, หญิงสาวฉีดสเปิร์ม แพทย์ค้านป่องไร้สามี, 'Ladies Inject Sperm. Doctors Oppose Pregnancy without Husband.'

32. *Thai Rath,* 2 November 2001, 'Five Famous Hospitals Trading Eggs and Sperms.'
33. *Thai Rath,* 31 October 2001, 'Beware of Danger. Females Sell Eggs, Males Sell Sperms. Openly Trade at Many Hospitals. Foreigners Rush to Buy!'
34. *BizWeek,* 15 May 2001, หมอไทยโชว์เงินหมื่นบาททำทารกจีเอ็ม, 'Thai Doctors Showed Off, 10,000 baht can Create GM Baby.'
35. *Bangkok Post,* 15 May 2001; *The Nation,* 15 May 2001.
36. *Matichon,* 6 August 1987, แนะออกกฎหมายคุมเด็กหลอดแก้ว ป้องกันหญิงรับจ้างตั้งท้อง, '(Doctors) Suggest Legislation Introduction to Monitor IVF and Prevent Commercial Surrogacy.'
37. *Bangkok Post,* 1 August 1997, 2, 'New Legislation to Safeguard Rights of Test Tube Babies.'
38. *Thai Post,* 27 May 2000, เด็กผสมเทียม-อุ้มบุญเจอปัญหาพัลวัน, 'Babies Born with ARTs and Surrogacy Faced with Confused Problems.'
39. *Matichon,* 27 May 2000, แพทยสภาชี้อุ้มบุญเริ่มมีปัญหาสังคม เผยปู่ย่าริบสมบัติไม่รับหลานหลอดแก้ว: the Medical Council of Thailand suggested that surrogacy has created social problems and revealed that 'grandparents have taken their property/heritage back, refusing to take test tube grandchild'. The cases described are of interest as all revolve around financial dealings and point to the salience of inheritance among elite business families in Thailand. The first involved civil servants of a university who requested reimbursement of their child's medical treatment fees and tuition fees. However, as this baby was born by using the husband's sperm and the wife's egg and a surrogate mother, it was ruled that the couple did not have the right to receive reimbursement, as they are not lawful parents of the child. In another case, a woman appealed that her husband's parents had promised that they would give their assets to any of their children who could give them a grandson. So she and her husband underwent assisted reproductive treatment and got a son. The husband's parents then gave her and her husband some land. Her husband later pledged this land as a mortgage in order to get money from the bank to run his business. However, after the grandparents knew that this child was born via ART, they didn't accept the child and recalled their land and assets. The husband consequently would no longer accept this child as his own and refused to look after the child. They eventually divorced. The final case cited in the newspaper report involved a woman whose husband wanted a son and asked her to get ART treatment using her egg and her husband's sperm. However, they did not understand that they could not choose the sex of the baby and the first and a second child produced were both girls. Her husband subsequently divorced her. The court ordered the husband to recognize and support the two girls as his children.
40. *Matichon,* 8 July 2001, 'Pushing Surrogate Baby Legislation: Problems with Rights, Concerns over Complicated Future.'

41. *Thai Rath,* 8 August 2005, 'Female Members of Parliament Pushed ART Legislation.'
42. *Thai Rath,* 23 February 2006, เตรียมยกร่างกม. ให้ 'อุ้มบุญ' ทารก, 'Prepare to Introduce Legislation – Allowing for Surrogacy.'
43. Nattaya Boonpakdee was quoted in the e-magazine *Samnakkhaw chao-baan,* 6 August 2008, 'Women's Health Advocacy Foundation claimed surrogacy legislation is unfair,' www.thaipeoplepress.com.
44. Similarly, the availability of social sex selection services through the use of preimplantation genetic diagnosis has become a popular service for foreign couples in Thailand (Whittaker 2012).
45. Bhagwati 2002 refers to 'rotten trade' as a trade in 'bads' such as arms, drugs, stolen goods, toxic products as well as the traffic in human beings and body parts.
46. The company is also known under the names 'Babe 101' or 'Baby 1001' which all go to the same website.
47. Anonymous, *The Nation,* 28 February 2011, 'Legal Opinion Sought on Doctors in Baby Trade.'
48. Prasert, P. *The Nation,* 25 July 2014, 'Sex-selection reports trigger investigation of fertility clinics.'
49. Murdoch, L. & Snow, D. *The Age,* 9 August 2014, 'Rising distaste about paid pregnancy as Thai government moves to shut down industry'.
50. Gecker, J. & Doksone, T. *Associated Press: Worldstream,* 2 September 2014, 'Surrogate offers clues into man with 16 babies.'
51. Anonymous, *Bangkok Post* 15 Jan 2015, 'Surrogacy doc indictment postponed'.
52. Examples of typical media coverage include Whiteman, H. *CNN Wire,* 4 August 2014, 'Surrogate mom vows to take care of ill twin 'abandoned' by parents' and Murdoch, l. *The Age,* 1 August 2014, 'Australian couple leaves down syndrome baby with Thai surrogate'.
53. See Murdoch 2014 above.
54. The Australian press was full of calls for a legislative response to ban international surrogacy by Australians, see for example, Ekman, K. E. *Weekend Australian,* 6 September 2014, 'Ban the baby trade before it grows any bigger', and Yaxley, L. *ABC News AM,* 9 October 2014, 'Calls for international surrogacy inquiry after revelations of another abandoned baby'.
55. Hawley, S. *ABC News* 20 Jan 2015, 'Baby Gammy, one-year-old at centre of Thai surrogacy scandal, granted Australian citizenship'.
56. Berkovic, N. *The Australian,* 4 September 2014, 'Police checks urged in surrogacy cases'.
57. Anonymous, *ABC News,* 29 November 2014, 'Thailand's parliament votes to ban commercial surrogacy industry'.

Chapter 2

INCOMPLETENESS

> Thai society may think it is something strange. I think when they hear the word 'test-tube baby' it is scary. It is like it is in a laboratory tube. Later on I think society will accept it. It doesn't mean they are against it or anything.... This is a kind of sickness that you have to get treatment for. It isn't something to be ashamed of. – Mon

Across the world, infertility is a source of intense social suffering and stigma. In many societies, the inability to bear a child is understood to reflect moral status. For women, failure to produce a child can be socially devastating, resulting in social avoidance to outright ostracism as they are excluded from social events and ceremonies (Inhorn 1994; Gerrits 2002). Women often bear the blame for infertility and may suffer physical and emotional abuse and abandonment (van Balen 2009; Inhorn 2009). For men, infertility is often conflated with a lack of virility and impotency, causing stigma and threatening their sense of masculinity (Lloyd 1996; Becker 2000). As Margarete Sandelowski (1991) and Gaylene Becker (2000) have noted, many infertile couples feel compelled to use assisted reproductive technologies to overcome their infertility.

The experience of infertility is relatively common. A meta-analysis of fertility studies suggests that approximately 9 per cent of couples across the world are infertile. Infertility is generally defined as twelve months or more of trying to conceive (Boivin et al. 2007).[1] The causes of infertility are complex and often multifactorial, including female and male factors (Zegers-Hochschild, Schwarze and Alam 2008). In some cases the causes are uncertain. Female factors include endometriosis, tubal damage due to sexually transmitted infections, and other iatrogenic infections or infections after birth or abortions, as well as a range of ovulatory and endocrinological and uterine factors (Healy, Trounson and Andrersen 1994). For men, a variety of factors cause infertility through the absence of sperm, abnormal motility or structure of sperm, or low sperm counts. Infertility increases with aging. Demographic changes such as later ages of marriage and delayed childbearing and other factors such as obesity also contribute to fertility difficulties and the demand for access to assisted reproductive technologies (Zegers-Hochschild, Schwarze and Alam 2008).

This chapter describes social understandings of infertility in Thailand and the experiences of the women and men of this study upon discovering their infertility. In doing so it sets the context for understanding people's decisions to utilize assisted reproductive technologies. In the first part of this chapter I describe Thai ethnogynecological understandings of fertility and the social value of children. I then describe people's reactions to the discovery of their infertility and the social stigma they experience.

The Stigma of Infertility

Infertility threatens gendered identities for women and men, particularly in Asian societies that place high values upon reproduction and where motherhood and fatherhood are considered fundamental to full adult femininity and masculinity. The sources of such stigma derive from the failure of infertile women and men to fulfil normative gender expectations.

Studies in East Asian societies influenced by Confucian values describe the strong cultural imperatives upon women to become mothers. For example, in China, women are often subjected to intense traditional and biomedical interventions to conceive (Farquhar 1991; Handwerker 1998, 2002). Despite the context of the one-child policy, Lisa Handwerker (1998) notes the aggressive treatment of infertile women and the social pressures upon women from family friends and work units to produce at least one child, preferably a boy to continue the patriline. Further, she describes the ways in which assisted reproductive technologies have become implicated within a 'new eugenics' in which doctors aim to produce 'perfect', genetically fit (male) children (2002). She demonstrates continuities between eugenics policies of the past and the use of assisted reproductive technologies now in China to promote the healthy development of an intelligent single child. In Vietnam, Melissa Pashigan (2002) notes that children are believed to bring family happiness and harmony between a husband and wife. Children are believed to bond families and build close ties between a wife and her in-laws. It ensures the continuation of the lineage and fulfils obligations of filial piety and the maintenance of worship of family ancestors. Women without children are considered pitiable.

Similarly, studies in strongly patriarchal societies of South Asia emphasize the low status of childless women. In Bangladesh, Papreen Nahar (2007) describes how childless rural women may be confined to their homes. For young urban slum dwellers in Bangladesh infertility results in divorce and desertion, with accusations of being worthless 'bad' women (Rashid 2007). In Sri Lanka the fertility of a husband is rarely questioned and a woman without children is seen as inauspicious and personally unfulfilled (McGilvray 1994). Likewise, among the Nayar of Southern India, Deborah Neff (1994: 477) notes that infertility is blamed upon women. They are deeply discredited and attempt to fashion new identities apart from motherhood, yet as Catherine Riessman (2000, 2002) notes, the ability to resist the stigmatization is class and age dependent, with poor women devalued in ways that affluent professional women may avoid.

There remain few studies within the diverse cultural contexts of Southeast Asia. In Indonesia, Linda Bennett (2012) describes how gender stereotypes blaming women for infertility dominate perceptions of infertility among medical professionals and are symptomatic of broader gender discrimination in Indonesian society. Among Hmong migrants to Australia, children, particularly sons, are viewed as the prosperity of the family essential to continue the lineage and ensure the reincarnation of parents. A woman who cannot produce a child faces marital insecurity and low social status (Liamputtong 2000, 2009; Nahar 2007).

Within Thailand, motherhood remains an important social status for women, partly due to the importance of the female line within the Thai bilateral kinship system. Adult status for women is conferred through enduring the suffering of pregnancy and the pains of childbirth and the many sacrifices entailed in being a mother and nurturing children (Whittaker 2000). Popular Buddhism celebrates an image of women as nurturers of men and religion (Keyes 1984; Kirsch 1985). This is taught both through religious texts describing such sacrifices and reinforced through everyday socialization and media imagery which reinforces an idea of the nurturing nature of women. 'Family' remains an important discourse throughout Asia, including Thailand. As Marjorie Muecke (1984) and others have argued, with modernization and industrialization the forms of female nurturing have changed away from having large families, towards providing education and wealth for their families; nevertheless, the social expectation remains strong that women will marry and produce a family and act as primary carer for that family.

For Thai couples, marriage is regarded as an intention to form a family and childbearing usually follows rapidly after marriage. It is assumed that couples will discontinue contraception soon after marriage. The failure to produce a child within the first few years of married life brings questions from in-laws and friends and exposes the intimate politics within women's relationships with their husbands, their families and society. Although there are increasing numbers of Thai couples choosing or accepting childlessness, particularly among the urban middle classes, such decisions remain uncommon and the very presence of these reproductive technologies may reinforce essentialized 'motherhood mandates' for women (Thompson 2002).

As a consequence, infertility carries considerable social stigma for men and women in Thai society. In my earlier ethnography on reproductive health in rural Northeastern Thailand I noted the social consequences of infertility for poor rural women (Whittaker 2000: 76–77). At that time in the early 1990s, assisted reproductive technologies were not well known and certainly were beyond the reach of rural farmers. At that time, my husband and I were also childless, a status which as a young, healthy couple who had been married for a number of years was not socially acceptable. We came to experience firsthand the constant intrusive questions, comments and jokes from villagers about our childlessness. I was urged not to stay on contraception for too long or else it would make me permanently infertile. Villagers openly questioned my husband's potency and urged him to eat raw meat and sesame seeds. I heard one man joke to another childless woman that she should *long khaek* – invite village men to contribute their labour by sleeping with her until she was pregnant – a reference to the communal practice of sharing agricultural labour among villagers. It was a joke she had clearly heard before.

Pimpawun Boonmongkon (1997) examines the social stigma attached to infertility and the pain and loss felt by thirteen infertile Thai women. She suggests that infertility causes a prolonged state of crisis throughout a woman's life. Women generally carry the blame for infertility. Thai society assumes that people will not have difficulty conceiving, so when a woman fails to conceive, she faces accusations of being a sinful person with poor karma, of not trying or wanting a child hard enough and fears desertion by her husband. She suggests three stages can be distinguished across a woman's life. The first is a stage of stress, sadness and shame when a woman first realizes she may be infertile. After this, women may seek explanations for their fertility, going through a range of diagnostic procedures and treatment, including the use of herbal remedies and religious pilgrimages. In the third stage some women gain a new moral identity, overcoming the dominant social discourses which define them as failures through several coping strategies. These include the incorporation of religious explanations of karma to interpret their suffering and childlessness, the redirection of energy into work and careers, or the adoption of a child. Boonmongkon's study is limited in that it is based only upon a small number of interviews solely with women. However, her findings are similar to another study by Kangsadan Chaw-wattanakun (2004). In a study of ten women seeking treatment within an infertility clinic, Chaw-wattanakum notes the importance of mothering to the status of women, with a number of her informants believing that having a baby was necessary for a woman. A woman's value is linked to her ability to fulfil four roles as daughter, working woman, wife and mother. Women tended to be the focus of all recommendations to the infertile couple. When treatments fail, people question a woman's behaviours, ability and desire to have children. This has psychological effects as well as affecting couples and familial relationships. The women in her study feared being abandoned by their husbands. Chaw-wattanakun (2004) notes the ideology of the importance of a 'warm' family in Thailand and the belief that children make a couple 'complete'. She found that women for whom treatments had failed tended to revise their definitions of women's identity, emphasizing their roles as good daughters and good wives.

Other Thai studies from a variety of disciplines document the social and psychological toll of infertility. Piyawan Sreeyamart (2004) utilized a questionnaire survey on perceptions and coping behaviours among 108 infertile couples at Srinagarind Hospital, in the northeastern region of Khon Kaen. She found that couples tended to keep details of their treatment within the family as it was perceived as a source of shame and they found most social support within the family. Men felt the need for privacy about their treatment especially because they feared perceptions that they were impotent and as a result discussed their treatment with fewer people than women. Other research attests to the distress experienced by infertile couples. A study of eighty women attending a northern infertility clinic has noted the feelings of powerlessness experienced by infertile women (Srivichai 2001). Studies suggest mental health among infertile couples is poor, with one 1992 Thai study finding 46 per cent of infertile people suffering from anxiety and 17 per cent depression (Anatavuthikanon 1992).

Golden Chains: The Value of Children and Parenting

In Thailand children are understood to bind the relationship of a married couple together and ensure the continuation of the family line across generations. The value of children in Thai society has changed considerably in the last two generations. In the past, as I noted in my ethnography of a rural agricultural community in Northeast Thailand (Whittaker 2000), having many children was considered important for the provision of labour on the family farm. The state-sponsored family planning program combined with the increasing costs of educating children and smaller landholdings has changed the desired number of children. A two-child family is now the ideal desired normative family size. But despite the smaller family norm, or perhaps because of it, children are highly valued in Thai society. Children are said to bring great joy to a home and are spoken of with great affection. Media and public discourse is filled with imagery depicting happy children within prosperous middle class families, reinforcing the trend towards small family sizes and an ideology of 'warm' family values.

Because many previous studies of new reproductive technologies have tended to critique the patriarchal imperative for motherhood, they have sometimes failed to acknowledge the agency, strong desires and eagerness to birth and nurture children motivating many couples (van Balen and Inhorn 2002: 8). Although it is important not to stereotype all infertile women and men as 'desperate' in their quest for a child (Franklin 1990), it is true that many of the women and couples interviewed for this study expressed steadfast determination to pursue whatever intervention available in order to have a child and their stories frequently involve lengthy medical histories of care seeking, religious pilgrimage, surgeries and multiple arduous IVF cycles. Many used the term *thamjai*, 'resolved', to describe their determination to continue until all options or their finances were exhausted.

When asked about why they wanted children, couples overwhelmingly stated that children make a family and their life sombun (สมบูรณ์), meaning to be perfect, complete, whole. By implication, women and men felt themselves to be 'incomplete' without a child. 'Incompleteness', *mai sombun*, is also a term used to describe disability in Thailand and reflects understandings of infertility as a reflection of imperfect bodies but also a spoiled social identity. This notion of completeness was the most common response to questions about the meanings of children or parenthood and indicates a view of childbearing as a source of self-fulfilment and fulfilment of a marriage. Having a child was viewed as consolidating and affirming the relationships between a husband and wife. Descriptions of a child as a 'golden chain' linking a man and wife were used. As Manit stated: 'People with families have responsibilities, a house and assets. A golden chain to fulfil your life.' His wife Nut stated: '[Motherhood] means a lot to me. I devote all of my life to the baby. Being a woman, I want to know what being a mother is like. I want to know how hard it was for my mom to have me. I have a perfect marriage but it's still not 100 per cent complete. I feel that another 20 per cent is from having our baby. Today, we feel almost completed. We only wait to see the baby's face, and knowing that the baby is healthy.'

The other term associated with parenthood was *rabichop*, 'responsibility'. Having children was described as involving responsibilities that signify one's maturity and provide an aim to life and self-actualization. For example, Pui suggested that 'perhaps having a baby makes us more mature. To look after another person. To consolidate the family. Because when you are without children you can do whatever you like.' This reflects understandings of bearing children as a marker of full adult status for women and men. Couples indicated that they were 'ready' for these responsibilities. The concept of *prom*, readiness, for children involves a sense of a couple having the emotional, social and financial resources to nurture children. Middle class definitions of 'readiness' usually include ownership of a house or apartment, the completion of education and secure employment. Phen noted that she had delayed trying to fall pregnant because she and her husband had not felt 'ready', only to discover that this delay had had negative consequences for their fertility. Phen stated: 'Now I think I am ready to raise a baby if we have one, now we are ready. We didn't think about it seriously before because we weren't ready.'

Children were also described as important sources of companionship and support to their parents in old age. This is consistent with the Thai concept of *bunkhun* – the debt of gratitude a child has for his or her parents which is repaid through meritorious acts by children that accrue merit for their parents during their lifetime. Filial obligations include support and care for one's elderly parents and people feared the loneliness of old age without children to care for them. For example, Phen said: 'I think if I have a baby it will complete [me / my life] and I'm afraid that when I am old I will have no companion because siblings are just siblings, but if we have a baby then the baby will be our companion until we are old.'

Linked to this is the importance placed upon continuation of the family. Despite the fact that Thai society is generally considered by anthropologists to be bilateral with traditions of matrilineal inheritance in the north and northeast, under Thai family law children carry their father's name unless the father is unknown. As will be discussed later, in this study men in particular spoke of having children to carry on the family name and 'bloodline' and inherit family wealth. This was especially the case for informants from wealthy urban Sino-Thai families, who emphasized the pressure placed upon them by their families to have at least one son to continue the patriline.

All men interviewed described fatherhood in terms of a demonstration of male maturity and responsibility. For example, contemplating his forthcoming fatherhood, Khiat said: 'I think being a dad and having a completed family (have changed me). I used to love going out and having fun. Since I have become a dad, I tell myself that I will never know the word 'tired'. I will fight for my wife and my kid. At the moment, I have not planned anything too far away; I just want a healthy baby and aim to be responsible for the baby.'

Ton likewise described fatherhood in terms of providing for his child: 'No matter what with mom or dad, the most important thing is that we are the ones who gave them lives and we want to give them the best we can provide.'

Although some men claimed that having a child was more important to their wife than to themselves, many women claimed to be undergoing IVF for their husband's sake. Pui described how her husband cried to ask her to undertake IVF: 'He really, really wants to be a father. At first he told me to do it. And I said "No". He was disappointed and he cried because he wants to have a baby. He said that having a baby has a lot of meaning for him. He is trying fully.'

Understandings of Infertility

A multiplicity of healing philosophies and array of etiological diagnostic and therapeutic beliefs around infertility are practiced by infertile people across the world (Inhorn 1994, 2000: 156). Beliefs about procreation influence attitudes towards infertility and infertility treatments (van Balen 2009). Apart from the relatively recent arrival of biomedical models of infertility, many cultures hold 'personalistic' models of infertility in which the inability to conceive is attributed to the actions of an external agent acting upon the women or couple such as ghosts, spirits or other people. In addition, 'naturalistic' models of infertility attribute causality to other factors such as humoral imbalance, or not eating appropriate foods (van Balen 2009: 37).

Thais resort to their rich pluralistic medical system to respond to bodily disorders. People who have difficulty conceiving resort to a variety of herbal remedies, appeals to supernatural forces, Chinese medicines and dietary interventions consistent with local understandings of the workings of the body and the processes of conception. These ethnogynecological understandings are combined with biomedical understandings of female anatomy and physiology. Hence it is not contradictory for women to be acting to restore humoral balance, taking herbal tonics, or visiting sacred shrines at the same time as they resort to high-tech assisted reproduction (see also Nahar et al. 2000 in Bangladesh; Liamputtong 2000 among Hmong).

In Thailand fertility is associated with a 'strong', humorally balanced body. In women health and fertility is indicated by regular menstruation that expels bad blood out of a woman's body. Abnormal menstruation is a cause of concern as it is understood to be associated with the circulation of 'bad blood'. Menstrual blood may affect a variety of organs in a woman's body and is contaminating and potentially dangerous to her health if allowed to accumulate in her body (Whittaker 2000, 2004). Physical discomfort during menstruation is associated with the 'bad blood' moving around the body causing a humorally 'hot' state. Headaches, 'high blood pressure' and fevers can all be indicators that this bad blood has moved upwards towards the head rather than be expelled. Women commonly consume humorally 'hot' *yaa satri* (women's medicines) said to 'bring the blood down' and restore the humoral balance of the body. During menstruation women also tend to take care not to disrupt the humoral balance, for instance, drinking cold ice drinks or humorally 'cold' foods are usually avoided. Sometimes 'bad blood' becomes dry, forming a lump which lodges in her womb, abdomen or backbone, becoming *phit* (poison) causing pain and potentially affecting fertility. Likewise, the presence of too much white discharge, understood to be white blood, indicates a dirty, cold womb and possible infertility requiring intervention through heating the womb. 'Mother roasting', the practice of heating the womb and body to balance the cold wet state of a woman's body following childbirth, is considered a prophylactic act ensuring continued fertility, sufficient breast milk and long-term health. Failure to follow this postpartum practice can result in the development of chronic pain, cancer and infertility. Likewise, abortion which is understood to disrupt the womb and cause imbalance as well as karmic demerit can also cause infertility.

Conception is traditionally understood to begin when the male and female fluids meet in the womb, blend and coalesce. Such a view is found in traditional medical texts such as the *Thai Book of Genesis (Khampee prathom chinda)* which describes the early stage of pregnancy as a delicate process: 'At the time of conception they say that [the embryo] is the finest particle, so fine … having been conceived in the mother's womb it can become liquefied more than seven times a day, it is so difficult to retain.… When the pregnancy has lasted seven days without miscarriage the blood becomes thicker, like water which has been used to wash meat. After another seven days it becomes flesh' (Mulholland 1989: 17). At some point in time this lump of blood receives the soul of a reincarnated being delivered by the ancestral spirits. At this point it begins to become formed and structured and animated.

Spiritual entities are also believed to directly affect infertility. During my fieldwork in a rural northeastern Thai village in the 1990s, infertility was sometimes believed to involve the intervention of spirits such as the *phi phrai,* a demon which eats the bodily discharges of childbirth. The spirits of miscarried children were understood to be capricious and may urge their siblings to remain with them in the spirit world, causing repeated miscarriages (Whittaker 2000). Some women who had suffered multiple miscarriages were understood to be cursed by a serpent spirit or *suang* which caused her to become a *mae kin luuk* – a 'mother who eats her children' – a graphic term indicating the stigma attached to infertility. An elaborate ceremonial 'killing' of the *suang* would be administered by a ritual specialist or *mor tham* (dharma doctor).

Before the widespread availability of modern pregnancy tests and visualization technologies such as ultrasounds, Thai women would consider the time when they could feel foetal movements as the confirmation of their status as pregnant – up until then the disruption to one's menstrual cycle was considered a sign of the presence of a mere lump of blood which may or may not develop into human form (Whittaker 2000). With the dissemination of reproductive technologies such as pregnancy testing, ultrasound and assisted reproduction, such embodied definitions of pregnancy and the foetus are being revised, yet, as will be seen in later chapters, early pregnancy is still understood as inherently ambiguous and fragile.

Although infertility is usually assumed to be a female problem, male infertility is recognized and understood to be either mechanistic in nature or caused through weakness of the body resulting in insufficient blood to form semen and insufficient strength to impregnate a woman. Like women, blood is important to male fertility and must be strengthened though appropriate 'hot' foods such as meat. Unlike women, male bodies are less subjected to humoral fluctuations and are considered 'closed', but nevertheless men are believed to lose vital strength through their semen. Things that affect men's humoral balance thus can affect their fertility. Intertwined with these understandings of male fertility, modern pressures, stress from work, environmental contamination and smoking are also said to affect the quality of male sperm and weaken his body.

Men's sexual function is commonly understood with a 'hydraulic model' of male sexual pressure demanding release (Ford and Kittisuksathit 1994). Unlike women's bodies which are understood to be open to outside forces because of menstruation and reproduction and hence inherently vulnerable and humorally unstable, men's bodies are perceived as 'closed' but potentially vulnerable when any substances leave the body such as semen (Irvine 1982). The fear of the penetration of the boundaries of the male body is well documented (Fordham 1998).[3] Masculine potency and hence strength is understood to be able to be affected by the ingestion of certain foods and love potions, and the practice of wearing *palad khik,* phallic amulets, is relatively common. These amulets protect the wearer against objects that might penetrate the body and divert spiritual attack but also serve to protect and enhance a man's virility and potency. Although many highly educated urban middle class men would not admit openly to such beliefs, the association between virility and fertility is pervasive in most people's understandings of men's bodies.

Discovery of Infertility

Every couple has a different story and set of circumstances leading them to infertility clinics. Most patients' narratives described complex medical histories involving a series of investigations and interventions before finally being defined as having medical problems. Many couples had waited many years before seeking treatment at an infertility clinic. Pook and Phen for instance waited five and six years respectively trying to become pregnant before seeking care. In some cases women who did seek care while still young were given fertility stimulants and no investigations. Although these treatments didn't work, a lack of follow-up care meant that the process of medical definition did not take place – blocked fallopian tubes and other problems were not detected and women spent many years trying to become pregnant to no avail before self-referring to seek further care. By the time they sought further treatment, their age and that of their partner meant that medical issues had usually become more complex, requiring high-tech interventions. As will be further discussed in chapter 8, men typically delayed seeking testing. Lek and her husband didn't think they were infertile, but that because of their age and busy working lives which kept them often apart, they saw their failure to become pregnant, despite not using contraception, as being due to circumstance and destiny rather than pathology:

> At first I thought I and my husband didn't have any problem I thought that it might be because [we are having a baby] late and we hardly slept together.... Since we were married we haven't used any contraception. We thought there would be no problem until our friend told us to go and check and so we did. We weren't busy then so I came with a friend and after the test we both had a problem.... [Our family] have waited anxiously since our second year of marriage. But we were stubborn thinking that we would wait and wait and wait. We thought that we could have our own. We thought that maybe the time hadn't come.

In this quote Lek describes the moment when their childlessness shifted from a social issue – a source of concern for their families – to a medical problem: 'after the test we both had a problem.' The testing defined their infertility as a medical problem, for which they can and should seek medical care. My interview with Jon and Daeng also occurred at the time they were starting to become defined medically. In response to my initial question asking when they realized they had an infertility problem, they denied they 'had a problem':

> Jon: It's not exactly a problem. We just wanted to have a baby soon after we got married. Until now, we have not been pregnant yet.
>
> Daeng: We are getting older.
>
> Jon: So we are afraid.

> Daeng: A year has gone by but why haven't we had a baby yet even though we are not on any form of contraceptives? We previously have gone to see a doctor at W Hospital. At W Hospital, we were told that everything was fine and normal so we gave it another try. The doctor there asked us to go in for IUI but we wanted to give it another year.... We passed all examinations. Yes. The only abnormality was that I ovulate too soon so we wanted to try ourselves first. But after a while we thought that we had better seriously look at seeing a doctor.

Jon and Daeng may fall into part of the infertile population for whom no clear medical causes can be found. What interests me is that they demonstrate the pathologization of their childlessness into a medical problem. Although initially resisting such a label, they describe their gradual submission to the medical gaze, and their own redefinition of their lack of a pregnancy as requiring medical care – 'seeing a doctor'.

Similarly, Pui did not consider that she had a 'problem' until medical testing revealed and defined it. She described 'not knowing' and 'not really being interested' at first despite having been married for six years without contraception. She then suffered health problems whereupon she discovered she had tuberculosis in her stomach. It was later discovered to have spread to her ovaries and she had to have surgery to have her left fallopian tube and ovary removed. Last year she tried to become pregnant only to be told that her right fallopian tube is 'blocked' and so now has started treatment using IVF.

Interestingly, only one informant mentioned sexually transmitted disease as a possible cause of infertility, despite the fact that such infections are a major cause of tubal damage and infertility in women and men. Ladda spoke of the shock when one doctor at a public hospital suggested that syphilis might be the cause of her infertility:

> I was told that I might have had syphilis. I was so mad and had a big argument with my husband, accusing him of having an affair. My husband was stunned and thought that we had had a check-up before the last year GIFT procedures and we were fine. My husband has been married with me since 1987 and never been out with prostitutes since. He did do that before we got married but is it possible for the syphilis to stay around from then? We don't have a clue about medical issues but if it was syphilis, why didn't the other doctor say anything and still went ahead with the procedures. We went back to the hospital, not to see a doctor. We went straight to their lab to get the result. They could see that we were very angry so they told us the result. It was nothing. We were so mad and asked to talk to the

> doctor. I think that he should not have made an assumption like that which it almost ruined our relationship. Luckily, we realized it before it had gone too far. The doctor claimed that there was no way for him to know if we were sleeping around and all my symptoms were right for the disease even though we have mentioned that we never slept around.

As in many societies, male infertility in Thailand is confused with impotency and as such carries considerable stigma for men. Lloyd (1996) has described this as a 'fertility-virility linkage'. Thai masculine stereotypes involve strong dimensions of virility and fertility evidenced through large families and multiple mistresses. The belief that fertility is linked with potency and male strength has been a barrier to the wide acceptance of vasectomy among men as they believe the removal of their fertility will make them impotent and weak with an inability to work hard (Whittaker 1998).

Such is the potential damage to men's sense of self that most men in this study kept their infertility private and only a few were willing to admit to their friends that they were the cause of couple's infertility. Wives were expected to remain quiet about their partners infertility and some even lied to family and friends about the source of problems, shouldering the blame for the couple's inability to conceive in public and thus maintaining the public 'face' of their husband. Similar protective representations or 'courtesy stigma' are reported by some Israeli women (Carmeli and Birenbaum-Carmeli 1994) and by Middle Eastern women partners (Inhorn 2004b).

Gae noted that her husband 'was embarrassed to sit here [at the clinic]. Above the entrance it [the sign] says "Infertility". He was embarrassed and afraid someone who knew him would pass by. He was scared that if people saw him there they would assume he was impotent.' Within Thailand, public appearances are very important. Hence for men, being seen publically at an infertility clinic itself can feel discrediting, a public admission of one's infertile status. Mon described the stigma felt by her husband even though she is the one having difficulty conceiving: 'Among men they say that you are useless if you can't make your wife pregnant. His male friends said: "Don't you have *nam yaa* [ability, not a man]?" And when my husband heard that he felt bad about this. But he is normal, he has nothing wrong with his semen. I have the problem.'

Men described their shock, feelings of frustration and sadness at learning of their male factor infertility. Khiat, who had discovered that he was infertile due to a previous mumps infection, said, 'I felt as if I fell off a cliff.' Some men were compelled to follow up with further tests at different clinics before accepting the diagnosis. Lek's husband was stressed to find out about his infertility:

> He thought, 'Why did he not have a child yet?' Even though his friends who were married in the same year have all got babies. He himself is strong. And his work involves social events as well but he doesn't drink, only socially. He doesn't really smoke. 'Why does he have this problem?' At first he wasn't brave enough to come and see a doctor because he couldn't take it. 'Why doesn't he as a man have it [sperm]?' Until he had a test in the lab which showed that there are some [sperms] he started to feel better, less stressed.

Men also expressed guilt upon finding out they were infertile. Somkhit felt a sense of failing to fulfil his role as a husband to provide a child: 'I have to accept the fact. I feel stressed that I let my wife down. She is married to me and she is 100 per cent ready but I could not get her pregnant because my sperms have poor motility.' Poy's husband was shocked at finding out about his infertility and was further appalled at the insensitive comment by a provincial doctor to his wife that she should just find another man to father a child.

Unlike women, none of the men interviewed spoke of their infertility in terms of their fate or karma. Rather, all described their infertility as a medical issue. Such medicalization allows for the normalization of infertility (Jackson and Cook 1999; Sandelowski and de Lacey 2002). For example, as an engineer, Ton expressed his faith in science. He stated that he knew of many men with fertility problems, and believed in 'cause and effect' explanations of his infertility. He believed environmental causes were to blame. Other men also linked Bangkok's environmental pollution or chemical exposures in industries as possible causal factors. Urban living in general along with class were evoked by Manit, who suggested, 'Villagers have babies easily, one at the beginning of the year, another one at the end of the year. But people living in urban areas have to go through so many procedures before they can have a baby.' In addition to environmental toxins and urban life, significant amounts of alcohol and tobacco are consumed by many men and stress was also considered particularly damaging to one's fertility.[4] By locating the causes of infertility in the very heart of masculine activities and socializing, such as drinking, smoking and hard and risky work, men avoided any suggestion that their infertility demonstrated they were less manly. It was their very performance of masculinity which was blamed for their infertility. For example, Somkhit associated his infertility with his job in mines and drinking: 'I used to drink heavily, had little sleep and worked so hard. I used to work in a mine in Pang-Nga, only had a shower four times in a month. Now, I accept that I get older and realize what all that has done to me. I did not think much of it before the test but once I have found out [about the infertility], I realized that I am not as young anymore.'

Pressures from Family

Most of the participants in this study had received moral and in some cases financial support from close family members while seeking infertility treatment. Most were discrete about their infertility, talking about it only with close family members; in a few cases they had not told anyone about their infertility or treatment. Several mentioned feeling pressure from their families to produce children and heirs, especially those within Sino-Thai business families. For example, Ploy described feeling pressure from her mother-in-law to undergo treatment even though her own mother opposed it:

> Initially, I thought that I really needed to get the IVF done because my mother-in-law really wants to have a grandchild. Whenever we go to visit her, she would complain that she felt embarrassed that she still does not have any grandchildren. Other people she knows already have grandchildren not long after their kids got married. She kept asking me when I would get the treatment. She offered to help if we have problems with money. I thought that we could afford the cost of the injections but we won't be able to afford if it gets too expensive. ... I might borrow her money and then I can pay her back when I can earn money from work.... My mother did not want me to do this. She cannot see reasons why as it is costly and there is no 100 per cent guarantee that it would succeed. My family does not want me to go through the pain. I told them that I would be ok so they accepted it.

Ut and Khiat were bothered by constant questions over their lack of children and had only told Ut's sister and mother about their treatment:

> [We get] a lot of pressure, they constantly asked us questions. Nobody else knows apart from our families. Only my mother and my sister know. Others have no idea what our problem is. Wherever we go, people will question us about having a baby. It's also depressing whenever we see somebody else being pregnant, especially friends

> who got married after us. We got depressed and did not want to visit them and their newborn at hospital. Honestly, we couldn't accept it and cried. We felt that we were less than them. We have been fighting for this [a baby] each day.

Family and friends often gave advice to couples as to what to eat, herbal medicines to try, shrines to visit or clinics to attend. Some informants appreciated the support from family members, while for others surveillance by their families was a burden and constant reminder of their lack of children.

Attitudes towards Adoption

It is perhaps not surprising that among the participants in this study who were currently undergoing treatment, few were considering adoption as an alternative. In general among this group, attitudes were negative towards adoption, as it was considered inherently problematic. Many couples stated they had never and would never consider it. The reasons given for not adopting varied. Many couples doubted they would be able to fully love an adopted child. For example, Ut and Khiat stated: 'I feel that we would not be able to give them a 100 per cent of our love so I think it would be unfair for the child.' Adopted children were seen as problematic to raise and liable to grow up with feelings of inferiority and social problems. Bee and Pitak described themselves as scared to consider adoption because adopted children are a burden or difficult (*lambaak*): 'Because they aren't our children, if you bring them up and it doesn't turn out well this can be their vulnerability (*pom doi*) it is like a burden because it is not our child.' A common sentiment was that despite their upbringing adopted children would still revert to becoming like their biological parents and hence problematic. For example, Lek suggested: 'I have never thought about adoption. While we were raising a child he would be OK but when he grows up the blood in him which is not ours.... We don't know the background of the child, how his parents are, that's what I think.'

Men were especially averse to the thought of adopting a child. As will be discussed further in chapter 8, men emphasized the importance of having a biological child. One man quoted an old Thai saying that adoption was like 'eating another man's *miang*'. This refers to a traditional Thai snack food consisting of a betel leaf with tamarind sauce, coconut, chilli and lime which is created by an individual to his or her own taste. The implication is that an adopted child is of unknown quality and will be distasteful and unsatisfying to its parents as it is not their own child. For men of Chinese background, having a blood descendent was especially important. Laiat noted: 'My husband is the oldest son in a family with Chinese background, they would prefer to have a descendant from the same blood otherwise it would not mean much.'

Within Thailand couples have traditionally adopted children from within the family to raise as their own. This was described by informants as a more acceptable alternative to anonymous adopting. Although some informants had visited orphanages, they did so to donate money, food and toys to make merit. Aruth stated: 'I think that I'd adopt a child of my sister or a child of my brother. Yes, from someone close is better. For babies at the orphanage it is better to donate money.' Two couples had tried adopting nephews from within their family, but both regarded this as a bad experience. Teranit and his wife had adopted their nephew when he was five and a half years old. They tried to raise him for a year and a half:

> His behaviour was unbearable. Taking the nephew we brought all of his problems and all of my wife's family as well. My wife's parents, parents of the nephew all together with us. I was ready to divorce. Because we took him in he started demanding things of us. He wasn't our child.... In the end I didn't want him and so he had to leave.... When we had problems and quarrelled with his parents they took their son back and now they ignore us and my wife stays by herself. ... When he left he took everything with him.

As will be discussed in chapter 8, the practice of adopting children from within the family has its parallels within gamete donation. Although for many couples donated ova and sperm were undesirable, they were considered more acceptable if they came from a close relative, such as a sister, a husband's father or husband's brother. Just as in adoption, it was considered that 'keeping it within the bloodline' would ensure the quality and biological relatedness of the child.

Conclusion

Infertility carries social stigma and is surrounded by secrecy within Thailand. For most people in this study, realization they had fertility difficulties was a gradual process. Following cessation of contraception, some couples had spent years trying to conceive before seeking treatment. As I describe in the next chapter, couples often seek care from a range of different sources, shrines and temples, herbalists, Chinese medicine practitioners, in addition to undergoing high-tech biomedical treatment. I describe how treatment trajectories were often disrupted by failure to find the correct specialist service, poor diagnosis and years trying less invasive techniques such as IUI only to find them ineffective. Seeking treatment from infertility clinics and undergoing IVF also continues to carry a level of stigmatization and misunderstanding, as Mon explains in the epigraph to this chapter. This is changing with increased publicity about IVF and knowledge about its procedures, but most couples are discrete about their treatment, telling only a trusted few about it.

Notes

1. Figures on infertility need to be treated with caution. Definitions of infertility used in epidemiological and demographic studies vary and researchers stress the implications of these variable definitions on quoted rates of infertility (Gurunath et al. 2011). For example, distinguishing between 'having unprotected intercourse' versus 'trying for a baby for a period of time' can alter the rates of infertility for a given population. Studies also vary their duration of time in their definitions: some use twelve months while others use two years. Gurunath et al. 2011 suggest a clinically relevant definition that accounts for maternal age and duration.
2. This idiom refers to a Buddhist idea of people as being links in a golden chain of love, in this case, love between a man and wife.
3. For example, in the shrinking penis scare of 1976, fears of communist Vietnam led to rumours claiming that the potency of Thai men was being destroyed through white powder being put into food. This led to an epidemic of men from Northern and Northeastern Thailand complaining of penile shrinkage and sexual impotence (Irvine 1982).
4. Factors such as traffic pollutants (De Rosa et al. 2003) and occupational exposure (Jensen, Bonde and Joffe 2006) as well as smoking are known to affect semen quality. Research into other sources of environmental contamination and its effects on fertility are ongoing. High blood mercury concentration is also associated with male and female infertility and high seafood consumption in other Southeast Asian countries such as Hong Kong has been noted to be associated with raised blood mercury concentrations (Choy et al. 2002).

Chapter 3

Begging for Babies

> We are Buddhist, it is common for us to ask or beg for a baby, Buddhists tend to leave their hopes with something you can't see. – Nut and Manit

The unpredictable nature of conception sometimes requires intervention by gods and doctors. In Thailand, infertility is viewed as a consequence of one's past deeds in previous lives, karma (*kaam*) and fate (*khro*) as much as a medical issue. As a result, couples experiencing fertility difficulties will implore a fertility pantheon for intervention in their quest to form a family at the same time as they undertake high-tech assisted reproductive treatment. Visiting shrines provides the opportunity for patients to be proactive agents in seeking care for their infertility, requesting, begging and bargaining for various forms of spiritual intervention on one's behalf.

In this chapter I consider the ways in which religion continues to play an important role in reproduction in Thailand, even within a select population committed to 'high-tech' interventions to cure their infertility. Syncretic medical practices complement pluralistic religious practices as couples pursue a range of treatments as well as a range of spiritual and religious interventions. To my surprise, the literature on health and reproduction in Thailand fails to describe the associations between shrines, pilgrimages and fertility. This chapter addresses this gap by describing a range of religious spaces in Thailand as forming part of a 'sacred geography of fertility' appealed to by infertile couples. I argue that these shrines have particular gendered significance for women in their pursuit of children.

They represent further examples of the intersection between the sacred and the ordinary, religion and magic in Thai society.

Although here I only discuss a few of the major sacred sites visited by the informants in my study, many such sites exist throughout Thailand. These journeys speak not only of the intense desire of couples for children, but the array of locations reflects the diversity of Thai religious belief and practice. I discuss the inter-relationship between religion and fertility and how these shrines offer people (particularly women) a means to intervene in the supernatural world without the mediation of (male) monks.

In many ways, such pilgrimages in the spiritual realm have their own parallels in treatment seeking within the biomedical realm. Both involve syncretic care seeking at multiple sites, both are enveloped by a sense of enchantment and appeal to various sources of authority. Bharadwaj (2006b) writes of the 'sacred modernity' evident in the laboratory practices and clinical spaces of assisted reproduction. In Indian infertility clinics he describes the creative continuities between the Hindu worldview and clinical practices and understandings. Uncertain and failed outcomes are explained by the role of destiny and God and cosmic forces (Bharadwaj 2006a).

Ara Wilson (2008: 632) makes an important observation that magico-religious practices associated with shrines should be considered not as vestiges of 'traditional elements' of non-Western urbanity, but as equally modern expressions of religiosity. In the same way, we can view people's resort to shrines seeking care and cures – their approach to what we might call 'the fertility pantheon' – not as an archaic practice on an axis of tradition to modernity, but coeval spiritual practices coexisting with high technology treatments. These circuits through the 'sacred geography of healing/fertility' in Thailand are layered upon other spiritual quests. And as I later suggest in this chapter, there are a number of similarities in the ways both are deployed and experienced by infertile couples.

In doing so this chapter contributes to the anthropology of reproduction and to the study of religious practice in Thailand. Most studies of religious practices in Thailand have focused upon orthodox Buddhism, however there is growing consideration of other spiritual domains (for example Jackson 1999a, 1999b; Morris 2000; Kitiarsa 2007; Keyes 2006; Nilsen 2011). Pattana Kitiarsa (2005), for example, provides an overview of the 'hybridization' of Thai popular religion. However, with the exception of studies of the practices of shamans and spirit mediums (Golomb 1985; Heinze 1988; Morris 2000), the health motivations of visitors to shrines undertaking devotional activities has not been seriously studied. One possible explanation is that requesting health is such a ubiquitous part of people's activities at shrines that it seems unremarkable to commentators. The lack of this perspective within religious studies of Thai shrines also possibly reflects the gendered nature of academic writing on Thailand and religion (predominantly by men) in which issues of gender and reproduction have attracted little attention. And yet as I was to discover, a large network of sites is known and visited by couples seeking children, and a fertility economy of statues, offerings and advice revolves around them. Feeding local knowledge is the networking on the Internet which describes various people's success at various sites (see chapter 7). Taking these sites from the point of view of a woman or man seeking assistance with infertility reveals a 'sacred geography' (Wilson 2008) in which certain locations, statues and sites take precedence over others.

The Anthropology of Health Pilgrimage at Sacred Spaces

A range of studies in other countries document health seeking in temples or shrines. The most famous Christian site of healing is that of Lourdes. Wil Gesler (1996) describes how Lourdes is a 'therapeutic landscape' in which the physical and built environment, social conditions and cultural perceptions combine to produce a place conducive to healing. Similarly, the Buddhist shrine to Guanyin, the Goddess of Mercy, at Hangzhou in China is viewed as a 'transformative space, a space of becoming healthy and whole' (Walsh 2007). Other ethnographic studies at shrines primarily focus upon the role of religious sites in the treatment and management of mental health and psychiatric disorders (for example Pirani et al. 2008; Pfleiderer 1988; Raguram et al. 2002; Padmavati, Thara and Corin 2005) and the power of pilgrimage as a means of expressing personal traumas and loss (Nortemans 2007).

There are few studies of care seeking at shrines for infertility. In a study of women migrants and reproductive health in slums of Rajasthan, Maya Unnithan-Kumar (2003) mentions the use of spiritual healers by childless couples as a means of displacing the stigma of childlessness away from themselves. She notes that resorting to spiritual healers allows women to negotiate the usual control over their reproductive bodies by patrilineal kin and the state. In her rich ethnography of Egyptian women seeking cures for infertility, Inhorn (1994) details pilgrimages to various 'shrines of conception'; mosque-tombs of blessed *shaikhs* (Muslim saints) and Coptic Christian saints, and living spiritual healers. Women consider that the success of any treatment, whether biomedical or ethnogynecological is ultimately determined by divine intervention.

Victor Turner and Edith Turner suggest that journeys to expiate disease can be seen as 'rituals of affliction' (1978: 11) to propitiate those supernatural forces that create or perpetuate illness or misfortune. They suggest that such journeys are pilgrimages, rites of passage conducive to healing. Such pilgrimages are characterized by a period of separation from everyday social relationships. This is followed by a liminal phase when the pilgrim is 'betwixt and between'. The final phase involves a transition back to customary relationships but in a new state of being following the transformative experience of the pilgrimage (Turner and Turner 1978). Although sites of pilgrimage can be found anywhere, there is a tendency for many sites of pilgrimage to be in peripheral or isolated settings separated from the social political centres of society, in remote wild lands surrounding the 'ordered' social world. Utilizing the Turners' work, Erik Cohen (1992) described Thai shrines as either 'concentric' (towards the centre) and 'eccentric' (away from the centre) places of pilgrimage. He suggests a hierarchy of Thai shrines exists, describing 'formal politico-religious centres' such as Wat Phra Kaew (the Emerald Buddha) versus 'major' and 'minor peripheral pilgrimage centres'.

However, the visits to shrines and temples described in this chapter do not neatly fit into the classic notion of either a pilgrimage or a definitive hierarchy. Although some sites are located on the peripheries, away from the urban centre of Bangkok, in forest temples and obscure locations, many 'popular' sites are located within the city and most are easily visited despite Bangkok's traffic. Rather than involving a lengthy period of time, most are conducive to a short visit – compressed liminal periods away from the office or home. Visits to shrines to ask for children are purposeful but also generally considered *sanuk* 'fun', combining devotional practice with the touristic pleasure of an outing. Although visiting shrines to ask for babies carries some elements of pilgrimages, it is important to note how such journeys also form part of the everyday religious practice of Thais, in which it is common to stop to acknowledge a tutelary spirit, request assistance to pass exams, or divine lottery numbers conveyed in dreams. As James Taylor (2008: 21) reminds us, Buddhism in Thailand is best understood as a religious assemblage. Following Foucault, he suggests the question of religion might be viewed through the notion of 'heterotopias' – in which there is an eradication of accepted boundaries between the sacred and the ordinary in everyday life. This is beautifully illustrated by the dense and intermingled religious landscape in Bangkok as couples wanting children seek assistance from a range of gods overlapping their beliefs as Buddhists and their treatment as patients. As Marte Nilsen (2011: 1610) notes, paying respects and generosity to spirits is a fundamental moral value in Thailand and is seen to constitute a 'good act' which in turn brings karmic merit. Not only is respecting spirits morally appropriate, but it has a practical dimension; once asked to intervene, spirits can also become dangerous if not appropriately respected, causing misfortune, illness and even death. Visits to sacred places constitute the small quotidian acts of devotion and enchantment common to the management of everyday life, risks and concerns in Thailand and 'erase the line between religion and magic' (Nilsen 2011: 1625).

While not a perfect fit, I retain the use of the terms 'pilgrims' and 'pilgrimage' in this chapter as they capture something of the dedication and devotion with which people undertake their visits and the sense of transformation they experience. Not every visit involved asking for a child, some informants said they visited shrines for *kamlangjai* (confidence) and reassurance during their treatment. Such visits also reinforce the supplicants' status as moral subjects, who have done everything possible to improve their karmic status, propitiate wronged spirits or intervene in their fate. They allow people with fertility difficulties a degree of agency.

Nor is visiting a shrine an act of last resort or a rejection of modern biomedicine (Turner and Turner 1978: 22). Gesler (1996: 99) has described visiting Lourdes as 'a popular return to mystery at a time when the elite culture has turned to rational thought'. On the contrary, all the informants who visited shrines described in this chapter were patients undertaking high-tech modern assisted reproductive technologies to treat their infertility. Visiting shrines was not a last resort in a 'hierarchy of resort', it was simply another form of care and intervention described as a means to complement and enhance other forms of intervention.

Sacred Geography of Fertility

I adapt the term 'sacred geography' from the work of Ara Wilson (2008), who uses the term to describe her mapping of 'market shrines' – the small shrines found in workplaces, shops and market stalls in Thailand, propitiated by people to ensure business and financial success. As I discovered through this research on infertility and IVF, we might also speak of a rich 'sacred geography of health and fertility' that exists across Thailand – sites recognized for their efficacy in curing the ill or granting requests for children. They form integral parts of people's quests both as a supplement to other treatments and as separate interventions.

My informants in this study visited sites associated with the cults of Hindu gods and goddesses (particularly Brahma), Chinese deities popular within the Sino-Thai population, royal spirits such as King Chulalongkorn (Rama V), local guardian and tutelary spirits (see table 3.1). This diversity reflects the cosmopolitanism of the Bang-

TABLE 3.1. Sacred Places Visited by Informants in this Study to Ask for Babies

Theravadhan Temples/Shrines	**Locations**
Luang Phor Sathorn	Chachoengsao
Phra Tat Phanom	Nakhon Phanom
Phra Puttha Chinarat	Ayutthaya
Wat Phra Kaew	Bangkok
Nine temples in Suphanburi	Suphanburi
Local temples	Uthai Thani, Saraburi, Ayutthaya
Wat Paa lae lai	Kanchanaburi
Doi Suthep	Chiang Mai
Guardian Spirits	
Saan Taa Yai	Bangkok, Nakhon Ratchasima
Village spirit post	Home village, Mahasarakham
Jao Phor Lak Muang	Kamphaengphet
Jao Paa Khao Kaew	Chiag Mai
Maternal house spirits	Chiang Mai
Mae Thup Thim	Bangkok
Ya Mo	Nakhon Ratchasima
Chinese Deities	
Jao Phor Seua	
Jao Mae Kwan Im	Yaowarat, China
Jao Mae Soi Dok Maak	Ayutthaya
Brahman Statues	
Phra Prom	Bangkok
Phra Pickanet	Nakhon Prathom
Royal Spirits	
Rama V	Dusit, Bangkok
Statue of Prince Mahidol in front of hospital	Bangkok
Somdet Phra Naresuan Maharat	Kanchanaburi

kok population which draws upon groups from all over Thailand. The list of sites named by participants in this study in table 3.1 is by no means exhaustive. It reflects the geographical origins of the informants of this study dominated with sites in Bangkok with a few sites included from Northern and Northeast Thailand (Isan). There are many other such sites dotted across the country. Not all patients could recall all the sites they had visited. For example, Ladda claimed: 'My husband took me there. He told me the name but I forgot now. There were so many people paying respects and plenty of garlands. I think all the patients and their relatives went there to pay respect and got better. I just want a baby so I prayed and asked from everywhere. I don't even know who is who (among the deities)!'

Not all of the people in this study had visited shrines. Exceptions included one Christian woman, Tuk, and one Muslim couple, Bee and Piak, who did not undertake such pilgrimages but prayed. Thus when asked about whether they had visited sacred places, Tuk replied, 'I prayed with God inside my heart, but God hasn't answered my prayer yet.' Only two Buddhist informants were true sceptics about spiritual intervention in their infertility. Mai, a Thai expatriate who normally lives in Britain, stated, 'With all my respect, I just don't believe in this kind of thing', and Poy laughed when we asked about seeking assistance from sacred places, stating: 'We haven't been to any sacred places (laughed) because even when we have come to be treated by science it still hasn't been successful!' Apart from these, all other patients had undertaken some form of devotional act to ask for a baby.

Ut (age thirty-two) and Khiat (age thirty-one) were typical of my informants in that they have visited many shrines. They have prayed for babies at the San Taa Yai (Grandpa-Grandma shrine), the San Phra Phrom in Bangkok (Brahma Shrine, also known as the Erawan shrine), the Phra Pikanet (Ganesh shrine) shrine in Nakhon Prathom and the Rama V statue in Bangkok. They also bought a small statue of Phra Pikanet for their home and Khiat also wears an amulet of Kwan Im (*Guanyin*, Mahayana Goddess of Mercy) and has undertaken a vow to not eat meat on every Buddhist holy day. Ut suggested that their trips to the various shrines strengthened them mentally and spiritually. Buying the small statue of Phra Pikanet for their home was particularly efficacious – they attributed their successful pregnancy to his intervention shortly after purchasing the statue on their third attempt using TESE/ICSI. Now, Khiat added, they would have to redeem the various vows they had made. Apart from these pilgrimages, Ut and Khiat had also donated money to orphanages to make merit, made daily food offerings to Buddhist monks and transferred merit to ancestors by pouring water at the temple on Buddhist holy days: 'We did so many things because we were very depressed (about our infertility) and we would try anything that would help us.'

In addition to visits to sacred sites, as mentioned by Ut and Khiat, many women and men prayed for children at personal shrines at home, furnished with devotional objects and statues purchased from the many shops specializing in sacred items. Devotional practices such as meditation, periods of renunciation symbolized by wearing white and fasting would also be undertaken as offerings. In addition, amulets of particular deities, such as Kwan Im, were carried or worn by women and men. Lingam (*palad khik*), representing the phallus of Shiva, was also worn (usually) by men to enhance potency and fertility as well as for protection. Some versions considered appropriate for women to wear to enhance fertility are also available for purchase in markets and on the Internet. Ying also spoke of her visits to spirit mediums in the first years of her treatment in her quest to ask for a child. All such practices allow individuals access to sources of magico-religious power outside of formal Buddhist practice.

Individual pursuits of interventions by various spirits and deities at shrines might also be read as a resort to alternate powers outside of authorized Buddhism. Peter Jackson (1999b: 245) suggests contemporary 'postmodern' Buddhism in Thailand displays an increased emphasis on the supernatural as distinct from rationalist/doctrinal Buddhism which was associated with attempts to reform and institutionalize the Sangha as part of the project of Thai modernity. Likewise, Richard O'Connor (1993: 336) has suggested that magical forms of devotional practice are a response to the centralization of the governance of the Buddhist order which insisted on orthodoxy and removed 'curing and magical arts, denying the benevolent protective powers that brought people to the wat'.

Pilgrimages to sacred places must also be read within the context of the commodification of urban religiosity in Thailand (Jackson 1999a, 1999b; Wilson 2008). Overlapping these sites is a thriving commercial economy of tourist-oriented fairs, amulets, religious artefacts and markets. This is not unique to Thailand; for example, the famous shrine to Mary of Lourdes has distinct sacred and commercial zones, contrasting the silence of religious practices with the profane spaces of shops selling religious tourist souvenirs, hotels and restaurants (Gesler 1996: 102). Likewise, at nearly all the sites described here, a thriving market exists nearby, conveniently selling the items required for devotional acts, flowers, incense, 'sets' of items for particular requests, souvenirs, pictures, amulets and lottery tickets. Tourist companies offer special daytrips and package tours to famous sites, combining merit making with sightseeing and local delicacies. Similarly, a number of informants applied the logic of capitalism to their promises made to the gods and spirits, with emphasis being placed on the size and expense of their vows: one hundred boiled eggs, annual dance troupe performances, eight pigs' heads. While by no means as costly as IVF treatment, large expenditures were seen to improve one's chances of success.

To illustrate the complexity of these practices, in the following sections I explore some of the major sites noted by my informants. The 'fertility pantheon' of Thailand draws upon sacred figures and places related to Thai histories of flows of religions and peoples. These include examples from all the different types of sites – from temples to Chinese shrines, nature spirits and tutelary spirits, Hindu gods and Royal spirits. In this chapter I consider seven such sites: the temple of Luang Phor Sathorn, San Jao Phor Seua, Tao Mahaphrom or Erawan shrine, the Shrine to Mae Thup Thim in Nai Lert Park, Wat Mangorn Kamalawat, the statue of Ya Mo and the King Rama V statue.

Theravadhan Temples

The site that was most commonly described as efficacious by informants for asking for babies lies 75 kilometres away from Bangkok in the nearby industrial town of Chachoengsao – the temple of Luang Phor Sathorn. It is the shrine most often mentioned by my informants in this study. The temple is named after a Buddha image which is said to have floated into town on the river on which the temple is now located (Hong and Hong 1987: 27, cited in Cohen 1992). It is a popular pilgrimage centre with a steady flow of visitors, especially on weekends and festival days and has an extensive market across the road selling local delicacies, flowers and ritual objects, parking spaces, food and drinks, as well as tortoises and fish to be released in merit making by worshippers. The site is dominated by an impressive white 'new' Sothornvararamvoraviharn temple (see figure 3.1). Within its main hall, or *ubosot,* sits a group of Buddha statues, the most important of which is that of Luang Phor Sathorn, dressed in robes, the original statue now encased within a larger

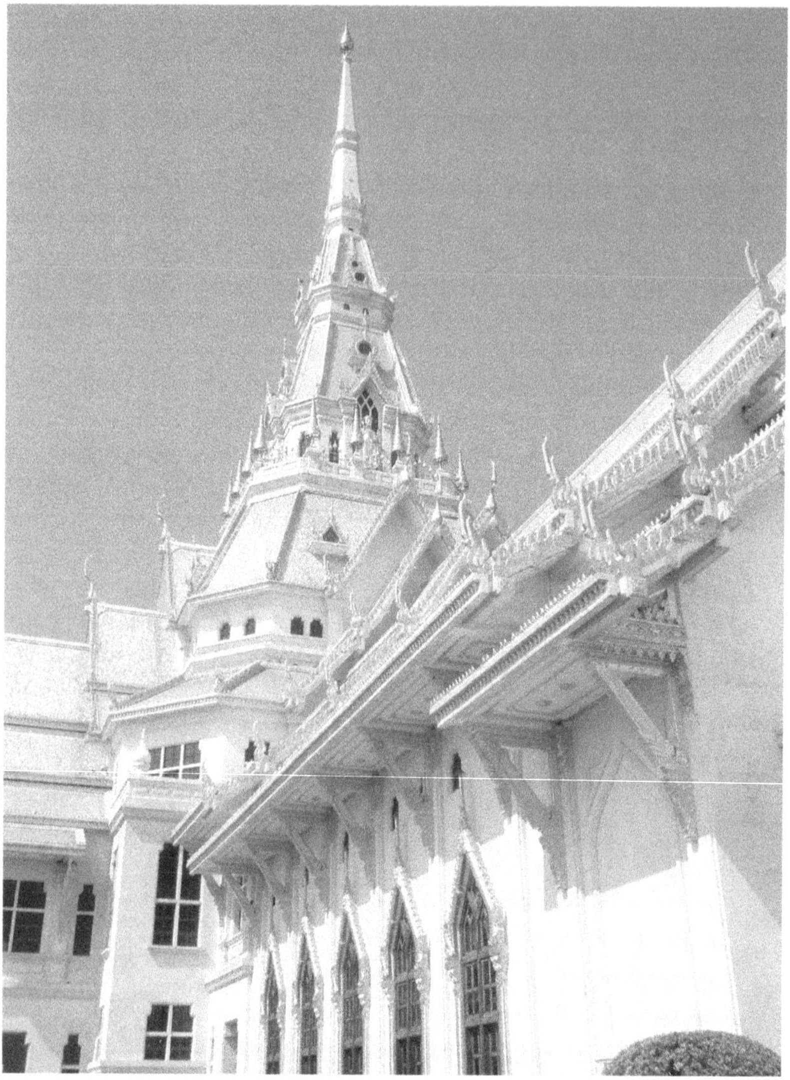

FIGURE 3.1. The 'new' *ubosot* of Luang Phor Sathorn.

gold statue and not directly accessible to worshippers. Votive offerings of candles, lotus flowers and incense are made and there are numerous collection boxes into which worshippers place money. The atmosphere is one of restrained formality.

The vast main hall has a multilevel roof rising like a *chedi,* and the eighth level contains a relic of Buddha and has four statues of Buddha facing four directions to important sites of the Buddhist world in China, Indonesia, Cambodia and India thereby linking this site with other places of pilgrimage. The floor of the temple is beautifully inlaid with images of fish, turtles and river life, harking back to the story of the discovery of the Luang Phor image floating in the river, brought ashore to this spot. The officiate told us that if people wanted a baby they could either simply offer up their pilgrimage as homage to Luang Phor and ask for a baby, or pray in front of the image for a baby and in return either ordain as a monk if you were a man or follow the eight precepts for fifteen days if you were a woman (figure 3.2). A flower seller at the site also suggested that offerings of eggs or bananas were appropriate for a baby and that you should eat a banana in front of the statue, however all such offerings seem to only take place at the 'old' site.

In stark contrast to this pristine 'new' temple, is the adjacent 'old' temple, which more resembles an old shed or large *sala,* hot with the crowd and smoky from incense. The 'new' temple took ten years to build. A temple officiate explained that because it took so long to build, some people are confused as to which is the original site and mistakenly believe the 'old' temple to be positioned on the original site.

Although it resembles a temporary structure, it continues to be visited by pilgrims. Unlike the 'new' temple, it is noisy and crammed

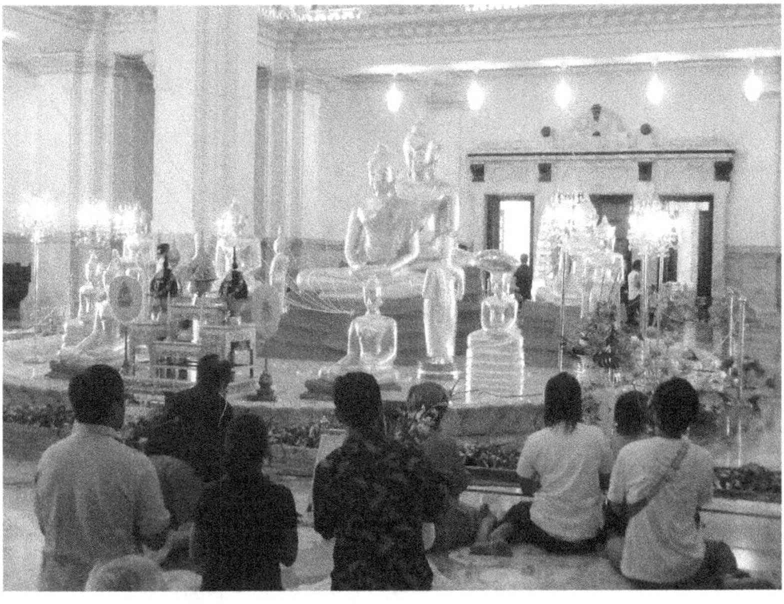

FIGURE 3.2. Praying to Luang Phor Sathorn at the 'new' site.

with worshippers, many of whom are offering huge piles of boiled eggs to a set of Buddha images which locals advised us include the 'real' image of Luang Phor Sathorn (see figure 3.3). Again in contrast to the 'new' temple, in the 'old' temple, the statues are directly accessible to worshippers who crowd inside to apply gold leaves to the image and make offerings of flowers. Towards the front of the 'old' hall, Thai classical dance troupes are available for supplicants to hire to make a votive offering, the number of dancers depending on the amount paid. Such dances are often offered in thanks for the granting of the supplicants' requests. The temple also offers other merit-making activities such as drinking lustral water. People also cast red *chensi* divination sticks to ask about their future or to request assistance from the *saksit* (magical power) of the principal Buddha statue. Some of those we spoke to said they were there seeking good luck (there are lottery ticket sellers plying their trade throughout the area) for children's examinations and to ask for a child. One woman told us: 'If successful you offer one hundred boiled eggs ... if your wish is granted your child will tend to be a dark-skinned boy and you may not hit the child or the boy may return [to Luang Phor].'

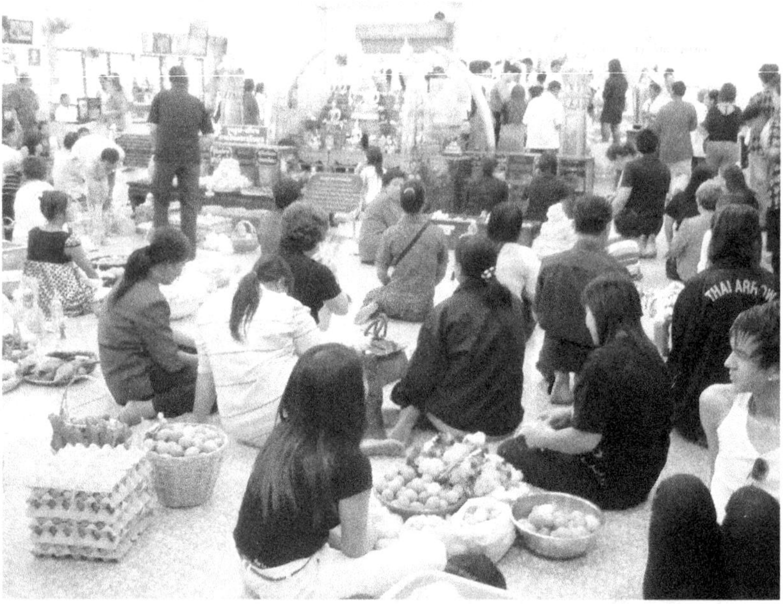

FIGURE 3.3. Making offerings at the 'old' site of Luang Phor Sathorn. The Buddha statues are in the background surrounded by pilgrims.

Mot, one of the women undertaking IVF, described how she had offered boiled eggs and a performance by the resident dance troupe at Wat Luang Phor Sathorn before both of her pregnancies. She and her husband had previously visited Wat Phra Kaew (the Emerald Buddha, considered one of the most sacred, meritorious and powerful sites in the Thai state), Phra Prom (the Erawan Bhrama shrine described below), shrines at the hospitals where they sought care and a shrine at Kasetsart University. But they were only successful after visiting Luang Phor Sathorn. She explained: 'We have been to both [the new and old temple] but we redeemed the vows at the old temple. I offered boiled eggs as well but we were told to offer the performances. We did and we got the babies! We still need to go to redeem the vow every year because people believe that the babies are His [Luang Phor's] babies.'

The Luang Phor Sathorn temple materially represents the tensions between institutionalized Buddhism and popular religion in Thailand. Erik Cohen (1992) suggests Thai pilgrimage sites fall into two categories, 'formal' or 'popular' sites. He describes the dominant motivation for the former category as the acquisition of Buddhist *bun* or merit, whilst pilgrimages to the latter sites are dominated by appeals for assistance from the concrete magical powers – *saksit* – of the image or person at the centre. Writing before the construction of the 'new' temple, he described Luang Phor Sathorn as a 'popular' site – 'a minor peripheral pilgrimage site' dominated by requests for *saksit* assistance. With the construction of the new temple, such a clear categorization between the formal and popular is no longer so easily made. Between the two sites, at Luang Phor Sathorn, the spatial representations and practices of an institutionalized formal Buddhist site now competes with the more magical 'old' site. The question of authenticity of the image hangs over the two sites as people move between the 'new' and 'old' sites and seek advice as to how they should behave. On one hand the 'new' site is associated with centralized orthodox Buddhist practice, charged with formal authority and stripped of its magical associations. People are advised by officiates to resort to orthodox means of making merit through donations and ordinations. On the other 'old' site people make their appeals directly to the highly accessible images, and are encouraged by their peers to bargain directly and make vows to fulfil their appeals. And yet the appeals are made to the same source of power, Luang Phor Sathorn. While religious practices may be labelled as 'other-worldly' or 'this-worldly' in orientation (Cohen 1992), the reality is far more complex and often fuses relationships with the divine with self-improvement, health and prosperity.

Such tension between 'merit making' and '*saksit* seeking' is also evident in other Theravadhan Buddhist temples. Although not as famous as Luang Phor Sathorn, many of my informants also visited a range of Theravadan Buddhist temples to both make merit and seek direct magical intervention. Most informants went to temples to accumulate merit to improve their karmic status, assuming that this was contributing to their childlessness. The sites visited break down Cohen's (1992) classification of some sites as 'formal political' sites versus 'popular'. For example, some this included visits to Wat Phra Kaew (the Emerald Buddha) within the Grand Palace, an especially auspicious and *saksit* image of the Buddha usually associated with the Thai nation. These visits also constitute tourist trips to '*pay thiaw*'. For example, Ladda had undertaken a merit-making tour featuring the 'Nine Temples in Suphanburi'.[1]

Apart from standard offerings such as incense, candles and flowers, offerings that symbolize fertility such as eggs and bananas (easy and prolific producers of fruit) or oranges (a Chinese symbol of prosperity) are common. Although as Ladda explained, in some cases the offerings take on strangely postmodern dimensions:

> I was told that I should offer eggs because I could not produce eggs and the eggs would symbolize eggs that are used in the procedures. The egg is a must. It might sound like I was mad but I went to Suphanburi to pay respect to nine temples. I was thinking that perhaps it was my sin that I had done something bad with someone without knowing it. That's why I could not have kids. I freed birds, fish and so on ... whatever I was told to do. At one of the nine temples I visited, I was told that the temple was effective to ask for a baby; anyone who came here, asking for a baby would succeed. There is a catch though ... they told me that the venerable monk there loves strange things. Someone came to ask for a baby and offered KFC chicken. The monk had no idea what KFC was but that person got a baby as wished. I went and did a similar thing by offering French fries. When I got the baby, I took French fries to redeem my vow.

As Ladda describes, appeals for babies are often transactional exchanges in which offerings are promised in exchange for success. Such activity is not described as merit making (*tham bun*) but rather described as *kae bon* (แก้บน) redeeming a vow. As will be described below, within Chinese temples, such exchanges also involve symbolic 'stealing' from the Gods – offerings given by other pilgrims are 'taken' and then returned twofold when a child is born.

Brahman Deities

Every day the famous Tao Mahaphrom or Erawan shrine (ศาลพระพรหม) at the Grand Hyatt Erawan Hotel at the Ratprasong intersection is crowded with devotees seeking wealth, success and power through their offerings and acts of devotion to the image of Phra Phrom (Brahma), a Hindu deity associated with acts of creation (figure 3.4). While much has been written about this shrine and its association with the prosperity religion of Thailand (Keyes 2006), it is also a prominent site for asking for children. The shrine was established in 1956 after a series of misfortunes and deaths of construction workers plagued the construction of the Union Thai Hotel. An astrologer who was consulted, Rear Admiral Luang Suvicharnpaad, had a vision that the construction needed to continue under the protection of Brahma (Majupuria 1987). The hotel was named the Erawan (after the three-headed elephant Airavata [Pali] upon whom Indra rides). The success of the hotel became linked to this statue. In 2006 a man said to be mentally ill destroyed the original statue of Brahma and was killed in retaliation by two bystanders. A replacement statue now graces the shrine. So significant is this shrine in the national imaginary that Charles Keyes (2006) has written of the ways in which the destruction of the image became

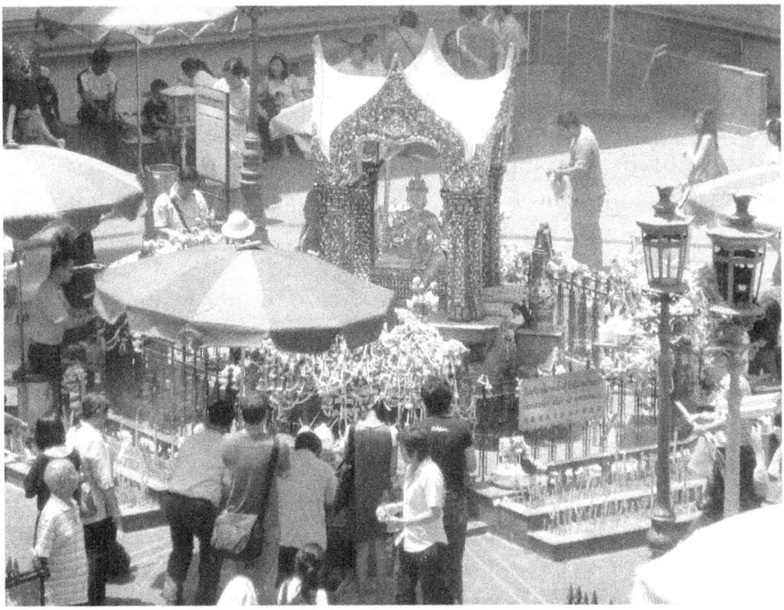

FIGURE 3.4. The Erawan shrine.

linked to national concerns about the Muslim insurgency in Southern Thailand and the legitimacy of the embattled former Prime Minister Thaksin Shinawatr.

Devotees offer flowers, garlands, incense and small wooden elephants and food offerings. A Thai dance troupe perform the *ram ke bon* (dance to fulfil one's vows) virtually nonstop at the shrine paid for by the devotees whose wishes have been granted. The dense clouds of incense smoke rise to the Bangkok Skytrain station walkway at Chitlom where passing pedestrians show reverence to the shrine by a discrete *wai* (placing their hands together and raising it to their heads). Lottery ticket sellers and large numbers of tourists add to the constant buzz of activity at the shrine.

Another Hindu God, the figure of Phra Pikanet (Ganesh, the 'remover of obstacles'), was also mentioned by some informants. Appeals were made to this figure to assist in the success of treatments. It was an appeal to Phra Pikanet that assisted Ut and Khiat in their successful pregnancies.

Chinese Deities

Given that many of the couples who attended the infertility clinics I studied were members of Bangkok's wealthy middle class and of Sino-Thai ancestry, it is no coincidence that Chinese temples were a common place to visit. This reflects the diverse religious influences across Thai history, and the more recent history of the acknowledgement and incorporation of ethnic Chinese and Indian populations into the Thai state. But it is important to note that resort to these sites did not necessarily follow ethnic lines, people who did not identify as Sino-Thai also visited Chinese temples.

San Jao Phor Seua (Lord Tiger Deity shrine) is a revered Taoist shrine built by the Teochew Chinese community in Bangkok and noted as a site for requesting babies by a number of my informants. When we visited in the middle of the afternoon, the shrine was noisy with a Chinese opera being performed in honour of the deity and crowded with people. The deity is tiger shaped and is believed to be the spirit of a tiger associated with the western cardinal direction who offers protections from evil.

Colourful stalls and shops surround this busy temple, filled with various materials required for offerings at the shrine. At the stalls surrounding the perimeter of the temple, shopkeepers advertise 'sets' of items for various requests, including the 'set for asking for a child' (see figures 3.5 and 3.6). Generally offerings are made of oranges, candles and incense and in some cases gold and silver paper is burnt. As some gods are vegetarian, offerings to those resident at the shrine vary; others such as the Tiger Lord prefer pork, eggs and sticky rice. A stall keeper explained that to ask for a child, a man should promise a sugar lion. These are beautiful elaborate moulded sugar figurines and are sold in a range of sizes (see figure 3.7). You 'steal' another person's lion and take it home. Another stallholder explained that once you take the lion home you can eat the sugar or cook with it or else release the rest into running water and then ask for the baby. After you have a baby you are obliged to return two lions so another person can 'steal' one. People requesting sons will steal a male lion, and if they want a daughter they will steal a female sugar lion. Once they have received their baby, they will return two sugar lions to the gods. An official informed us that the most auspicious day for asking for children is the fifteenth day of the first month (of the Chinese calendar). Apart from making offerings to the Lord Tiger Deity, this shrine also contains an image of Kwan Im and an image of Thai nature goddess, Mae Thup Thim, both associated with fertility.

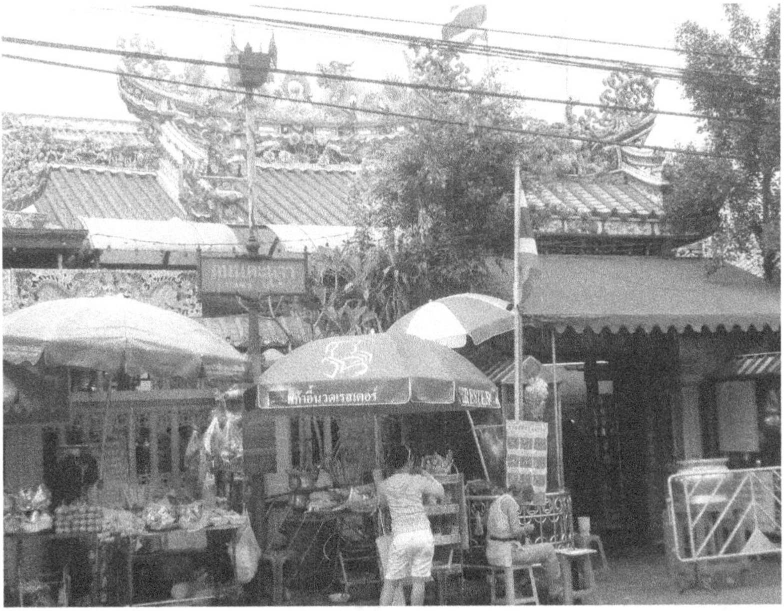

FIGURE 3.5. The entrance to Jao Phor Seua temple.

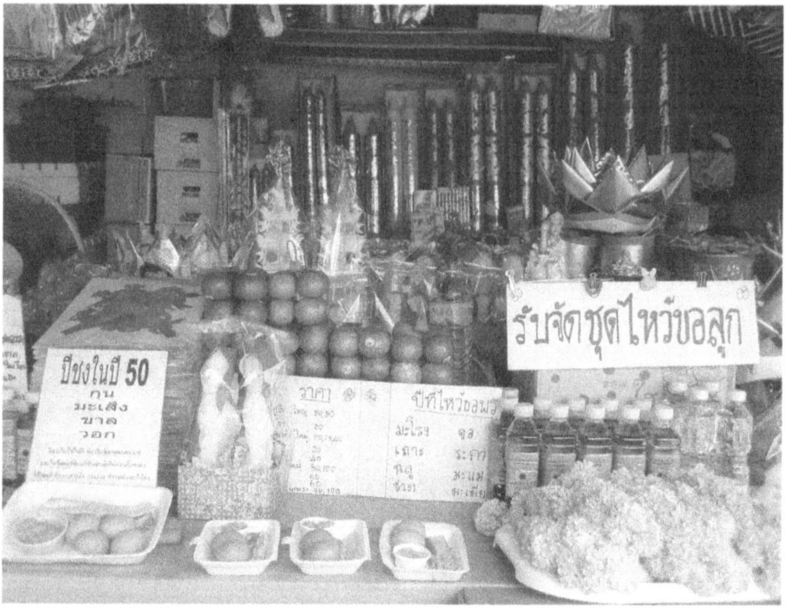

FIGURE 3.6. Items for purchase at a market stall near Jao Phor Seua shrine, including a sign advertising 'Sets for asking for a child'.

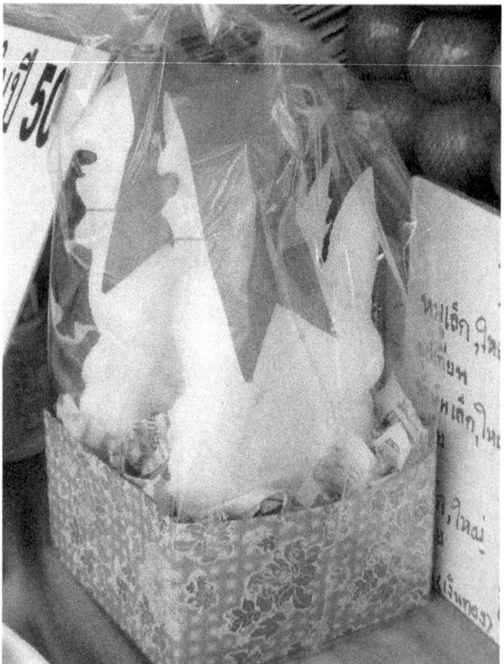

FIGURE 3.7. A 'set' of sugar lions for purchase to be presented to redeem vows at Jao Phor Seua shrine.

Stealing Oranges in Yaowarat

A further Chinese site associated with fertility is off the busy gold-selling strip of Yaowarat Road in Bangkok. Opposite the Talat Kao (Old Market) stands the Chinese temple Wat Mangorn Kamalawat (Dragon Lotus temple) but more commonly known by locals as Wat Leng Noei Yee (figure 3.8). It was built in the reign of King Rama V in 1871 by Phraya Chotikaratsetthi and was one of the largest Mahayana temples of that time.

This shrine highlights the religious hybridity of Thailand and the Chinese heritage of Bangkok. On either side, shops festooned in red and yellow paper lanterns, funeral paper goods, bags of oranges and a range of reliquary items line the street, the material culture and economy of rituals (figure 3.9). We interviewed two of the shop owners who are happy to advise their customers about appropriate offerings, rituals and auspicious times for offerings. Thinking my Thai research assistant Som had come to ask for a child, the first woman asked how old Som was and advised us that 'unless you are desperate, don't come here to ask for a child as the children who you ask for from the Gods are difficult to raise, "*liang yak*". You can't hit them or punish them or else they may return to the Gods.' The most appropriate day to come to ask for a child is the seventh day of the seventh month according to the Chinese calendar. She

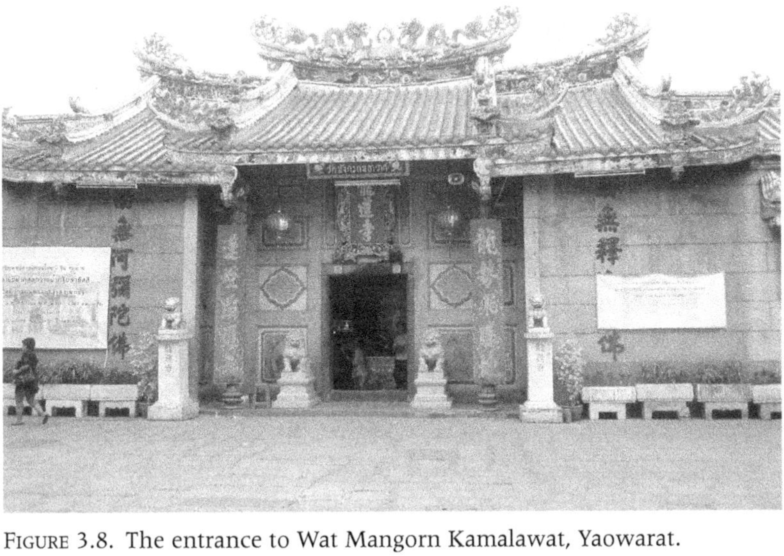

FIGURE 3.8. The entrance to Wat Mangorn Kamalawat, Yaowarat.

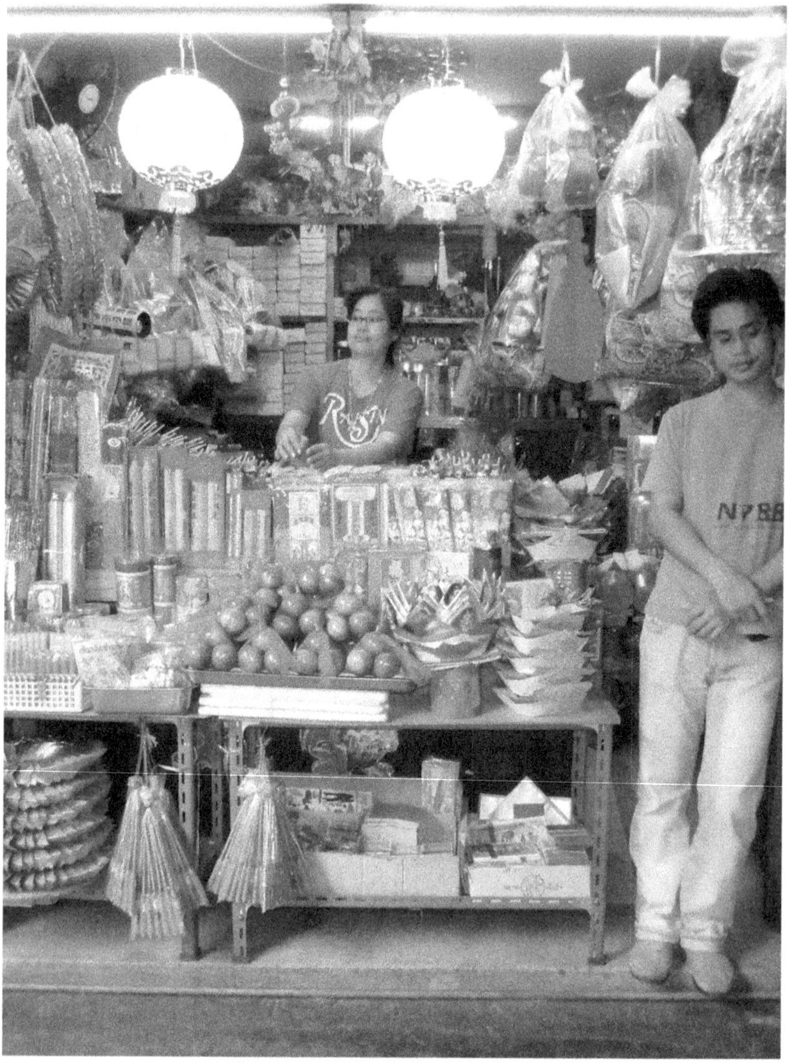

FIGURE 3.9. One of the many shops near the shrine selling religious paraphernalia for offerings. Note the bags of oranges for sale.

suggested that infertility had its origins in past incarnations: 'If you didn't have dependents (*borawaan*) in your past life then you may have difficulties in having children in this life.' She told us the story of a customer who came to the shrine and asked for a child from Kwan Im and the child ended up looking like one of her subordinates at work (the implication being there was a karmic link between them from a former life).

The temple entrance is overseen by four huge brass and polychrome protective guard demons. Once inside, a range of shrines, for fifty-eight deities, crowd the temple, each with its own area for placing incense and candles. Shoes are not removed, save for the immediate area in front of statues. No photos are allowed inside the shrine. Around twenty people, as well as a gaggle of tourists, were at the shrine when we were there. A constant stream of people moved in and out the temple. Many people light a large handful of incense and then place three sticks at the various statues, according to their prayers. The shrine is famous as a place to remove bad luck, *'sador khro'*, and to make offerings for one's children's success in education and exams. But it is also known as a place to ask for children, and in this two images are of special importance. The first is an image of the Bodhisattva Tao Mae Kwan Im, กวนอิม (the Thai name for Guanyin, the feminine form of the Bodhisattva Avalokitesvara), the Goddess of Mercy. There is a small brass statue approximately one foot high depicting her holding a baby, demonstrating her role in fertility. She is set in a glass case with nine other images of her in various poses. To ask for a child, one should make offerings of paper (a paper lotus or gold paper, later burnt at a small oven outside), incense, candles and oranges to the image. Oranges are a symbol of fertility for Chinese. You should then steal two oranges that have been offered by another person to take home with you. If your wish is granted and you have a child, you should bring ducks or fruit in return or whatever else you promised.

The other image sought by people asking for children is that of Mae Seu (the Thai name for Gong Phua or Mazu), another female deity depicted in a statue holding a child. The polychrome image of Mae Seu is about 3 feet high. Associated with the sea, she is understood by many lay people to be one of the many manifestations of Kwan Im and so also appealed to for granting children.

Guardian Spirits

Behind the white luxury of the Nai Lert Hotel, near the rubbish and service entrance, is a quiet glen mentioned in guidebooks as one of Bangkok's bizarre sights for tourists. It is an unlikely place of pilgrimage – a 40-metre-square site surrounded on one side by the service car park and on the other by a construction zone and neglected work area. The area around the shrine offers a sanctuary of shade and quiet. It is dark and atmospheric shaded by a large Banyan tree in the top left corner and other large trees, all sacred tress, as evidenced by the cloths tied around their trunks and the offerings at their bases – small models of *thewadaa* (angels) and attendants, candles, incense and flowers. In one corner of this space an old rusting filing cabinet sits ludicrously. I wonder how it came to be dumped there and what the pilgrims who come to this spot must think of the awkward juxtaposition of a sanctuary amidst the daily disorder and detritus of the service entrance. As you enter the site, you follow a path fenced on both sides by a row of small, multicoloured lingams. Some are carved from stone and many are red. I am struck by a beautiful red one which incorporates a woman's torso carved into the phallus trunk, at another's base is a small statue of a baby riding a rocking horse, the head now broken from the body but laid alongside (see figures 3.10, 3.11, 3.12). In the centre of the shrine is a small wooden spirit house, adorned with gold leaf on the right side, in front of which daily offerings of incense, candles, fruit and flower offerings of yellow marigolds and yellow chrysanthemums are placed by the hotel.

While we were there a woman from the hotel staff came to give the daily offering. Kneeling in front of the spirit house she paid homage for a short time and then arranged the offerings. She said many people still come to the shrine. Even his Royal Highness the Crown Prince had graced the shrine with a visit to pay respect, she told us. Thinking we had also come for that reason, she advised us that Mae Jao likes chrysanthemums and that offerings of fruit, incense and candles and a phallus are appropriate. 'If you asked you would be granted a boy child', she said. She said the hotel doesn't know how many people come, as no one counts. There was no particularly auspicious time or day to come. People simply came and asked and would return when they conceived a child to thank Mae Jao. We paid our respects and then I took some photographs. I was disturbed when the initial photographs did not work as though something was causing my digital camera to malfunction. Som suggested I should ask permission of Mae Jao before I took my pictures and explain my research to her. After doing so, my camera functioned perfectly (field notes 2008).

This shrine to the female deity known as San Jao Mae Thap Thim in Nai Lert Park is one of the more spectacular sites visited by Thais with fertility difficulties. While all the other sites described in this chapter are visited for various reasons, this site is solely associated with fertility. Couples seeking a child are recommended to bring a carved lingam, at least the length of an arm, to offer along with

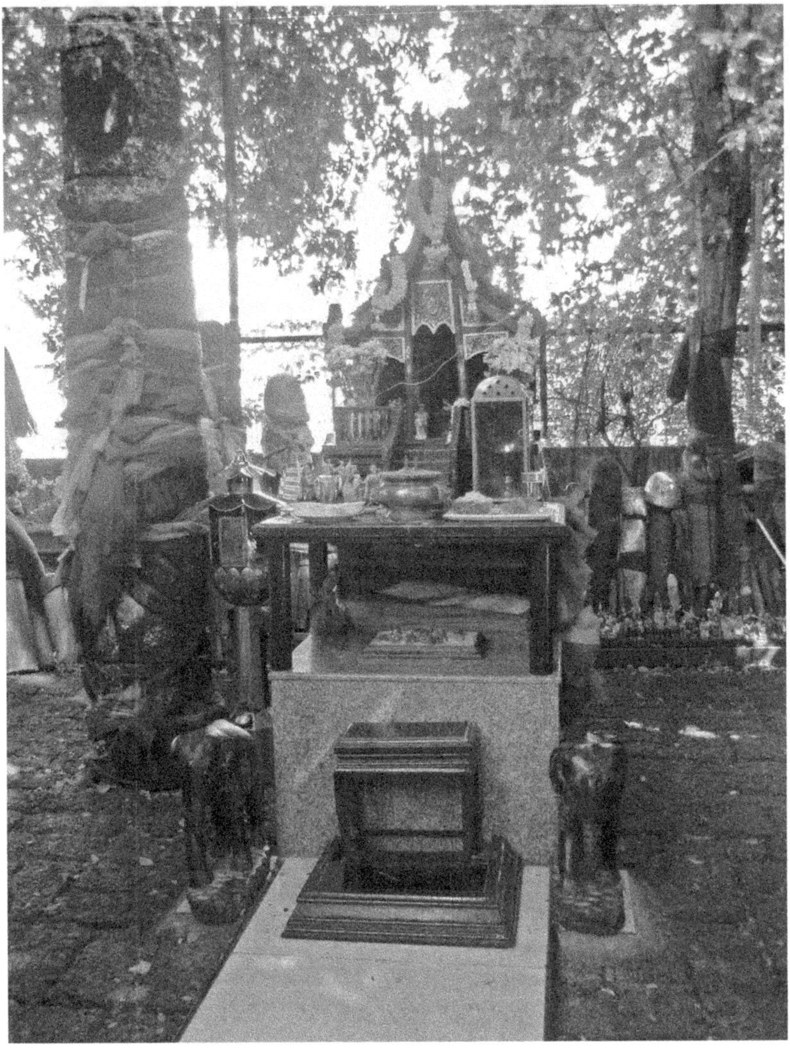

FIGURE 3.10. San Jao Mae Thap Thim in Nai Lert Park within a sacred grove, with offerings of flowers, candles and incense and lingams in the background.

food, a rice dish and dessert, and a standard set of offerings known as *khan haa,* incense, flowers and candles. Ideally, the husband of the woman seeking pregnancy should whittle the lingam offering himself, as it is the partner of the one who makes the phallus who will fall pregnant. A magic verse, *khataa,* is intoned during the offering. The shrine is said to have originally been built by the millionaire businessman Nai Lert, after whom the hotel and park is named, to

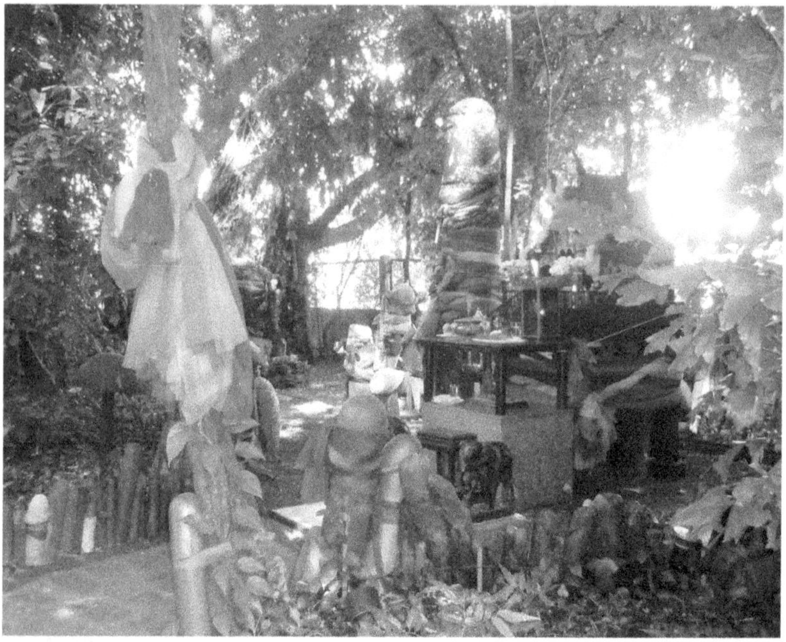

FIGURE 3.11. View of the shrine showing the many lingam offerings at the site.

honour the female diety said to inhabit the old ficus tree on the site. Shortly after the shrine was built, couples fell pregnant after visiting the site and a steady stream of pilgrims has come ever since. The deity Mae Thup Thim is a Thai female nature spirit associated with Banyan trees (which carry spiritual associations both with Buddha and the Trimurti of Brahma, Vishnu and Shiva). Her name, *thup thim* in Thai, translates both as 'pomegranate', a fruit symbolizing fertility, and 'ruby'. Phallic offerings are called *dokmai cao* (the flower of the spirit). It is clear when visiting the site that it continues to attract pilgrims; there are new lingams as well as countless older ones at the site. A small wooden plaque depicting Mae Thup Thim stands in the spirit house. This shrine thus merges together the representations of Shiva and beliefs in spirits of nature/protectors of places. She epitomizes the hybridity of Thai religious beliefs as a statue to her can also be found in some Chinese temples.

The Brave Lady

A bronze statue of Thao Suranari (ท้าวสุรนารี), most commonly known as Ya Mo (ย่าโม, Paternal Grandma Mo), stands in the centre of Nakhon Ratchasima (Khorat) city next to the Chumphon gate of

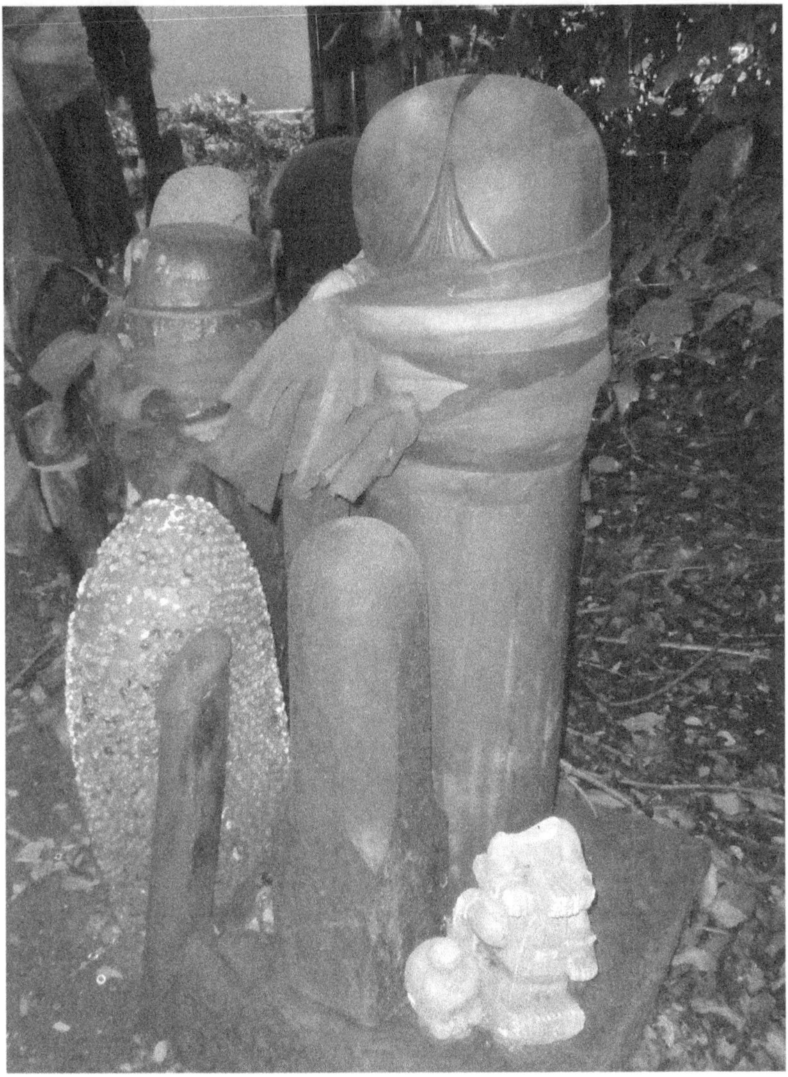

FIGURE 3.12. Detailed view of some of the lingam offerings at the site.

the old city walls. The monument was erected on 15 January 1934. The statue enshrines this northeastern guardian spirit who protects the people of the city. The story of this Khorat heroine is that in 1827 she fought against the rebellion of Jao Anuwong of Vientiane, who rebelled against the king of Siam. The people of Khorat were ordered to leave the city, but as the captives reached Phi Mai district, Ya Mo inspired the women and men of Khorat to fight against their captors and defeat them. Jao Anuwong had to withdraw; a Thai army was mobilized which eventually suppressed the rebellion and captured Jao Anuwong (Nilsen 2011: 1599). The title of Thao Suranarai (Brave Lady) was awarded to Ya Mo for her bravery by King Ram III. She is regarded as the grandmother/protective spirit of all the people of Khorat and stories associate her with cleverness, leadership, bravery, female charm and love of the northeast. The Ya Mo monument is considered very sacred *saksit* to local people, and her popularity is evident in the many people who come particularly early in the morning and at dusk offering flowers, incense, coconuts and fruits, foods, pigs' heads, eggs and other offerings. Despite her warrior strength Ya Mo is a benevolent spirit and may be asked for anything, but it is customary to give her a promise in return. For example, a common promise is to hire dancers to perform local singing and dancing *plaeng Khorat* in return for fulfilled wishes. A range of miracles are attributed to her intervention. Each March a festival is also held in her honour.

Despite evidence that the story of Thao Suranari was a fabrication associated with the Thai nationalist movement in the 1930s under Field Marshal Phibul Songkham (Keyes 2002), this has not dampened enthusiasm and belief in this figure, especially among the people of Khorat.

For her first pregnancy, Ladda had visited a number of sacred places, including Luang Phor Sathorn and the King Rama V monument, as well as the Kwan Im goddess in Yaowarat and the Chao Phor Seua (Lord Tiger Shrine): 'We had been to so many places. We don't even know where to go back to redeem the vows. The last place we went was Ya Mo [Grandma Mo]. I had asked for so many things from her and got them as I wished. I believe that she is real. At the time, I asked for one of her disciples to be born as my baby. Her disciples are soldiers so I was so sure that I would get a boy.'

At the time of our interview she had just returned from the Ya Mo monument where she had redeemed her vows by donating a dance troupe to perform and a hundred eggs: 'We went to redeem the vow at Ya Mo because we are very confident that she gave the baby to us'. She was pregnant with her second child for whom she had again sought assistance from Ya Mo: 'We offered her a dance show, betel nuts, betel leaves, coconuts and 100 eggs before I came to implant the embryos. I have been to ask from so many other places but failed every time. I prayed to Ya Mo to let whoever else [among the deities] that also helped us, know that all the offerings were for them, too.'

Female Deities and Spirits

Female spirits/deities such as those described above are important in people's quests for children. Although not mentioned by my informants, the Hindu Goddess Mariammam (Uma Devi or Shakti, Shiva's consort) is also associated with fertility. She and her sons (Phra Khantakuman or Subramaniam and Phra Phikanet or Ganesh) are worshipped at the important Tamil Sri Maha Mariammam temple (the Maha Uma Devi temple [วัดพระศรีมหาอุมาเทวี] or colloquially known less respectfully as wat khaek [วัดแขก] among Thais) in Silom in Bangkok. The images of femininity displayed by such figures ranges from the demure nurturing grace of Kwan Im through to the warrior strength of Ya Mo and the sexualized fecundity of nature spirits such as Mae Thup Thim. All represent sources of feminine *saksit* power unmediated by men.

Studies of Thai religious practice tend to consider gender only in association with debates within the Sangha about the ordination of women. In most studies of visits to shrines and urban religion (Jackson 1999b; Wilson 2008) little attention is paid to the gender of visitors and whether this affects their motivations and relationship with religious practice. However, in a study of European Marian pilgrimages by Christians and Muslims to three sites in Germany, Portugal and Turkey (Jansen and Kühl 2008: 296), the authors note that it is mostly women who partake in popular forms of religious expression such as visiting shrines. At these Marian sites women visit shrines seeking assistance from the female figure of Mary for intercession because she is a woman with the power to help them with violent marriages, custody disputes and family health matters. In her role as a maternal figure she is viewed as being able to mediate between sacred male relatives and common believers. Willy Jansen and Miecke Kühl (2008) suggest that as a feminine role model, the figure of Mary is more complex than often presented. The figure of Mary not only provides a gender script for women (her piety, purity and obedience as a believer and compassion) but is also imbued with courage and power. Devotion to Mary allows women to partake in forms and themes of expression often classified as feminine and enables women to circumvent religious authority represented by the male dominated experience of attending mass – a route to religious authority and direct paths to the supernatural without resort to mediation by men.

One might compare the figures of Ya Mo, Kwan Im and Mae Thup Thim with the Marian figures described by Jansen and Kühl

(2008). These are all strong and powerful yet accessible female figures who may act as intermediaries between the supernatural world and the mundane concerns of women. They are believed to have special compassion and affinity with women and understand their concerns. All are powerful, either through their association with fecund nature, spiritual achievement or strength in the face of adversity. Writing of Ya Mo, Nilsen (2011: 1623) suggests that such female figures 'each in their own way represent the love, goodness, virtue, compassion and selflessness of the Mother image' yet also female strength and endurance – qualities appealing to women undergoing the rigors of IVF treatment.

Royal Spirits

The pantheon of spirits appealed to by people wanting a baby include a number of Royal spirits. Devotion to the spirit of King Rama V (King Chulalongkorn, r. 1868–1910) became very popular during the 1990s, particularly among the Thai urban middle class. King Rama V is revered by the Thai nation as the king who is said to have created the modern nation-state of Thailand and protected Thailand from European colonization. It is common to see photographs and images of him in offices and homes, and amulets bearing his image are very popular. Reverence for King Rama V thus links expressions of Thai nationalism with desires for personal prosperity, but his image is also mentioned as *saksit* for people seeking success in their fertility treatment. Devotional acts of piety are displayed at the large bronze equestrian statue of King Rama V in front of the parliament building in the centre of the Royal Plaza in Bangkok. Devotees offer flowers, candles, incense and bottles of Thai whiskey each Tuesday evening (the day of his birth). It is not entirely clear why some ask the spirit of King Rama V for children, other than the belief in the sacred *saksit* power he manifests to overcome all forms of difficulties, a general parallel between prosperity (the multiplication of wealth) and fecundity or possibly due to the fact that in his lifetime he fathered seventy-seven children to his four wives and many concubines.

Homage is also paid to the statue of another royal spirit, that of Prince Mahidol Adulyadej, Prince of Songkla and father of the present king of Thailand. Prince Mahidol trained in public health from Harvard University and supported the training and dissemination of modern medicine in Thailand. The Royal Medical School later became the present Faculty of Medicine at Siriraj hospital. It is common practice for patients and staff at this hospital to pay homage to his spirit during their care there.[2]

The Dangers of Asking from the Gods

Requesting babies at shrines has its dangers. For example, the old shrine built on the remains of a Khmer temple site, San Phra Kaan in Lopburi, is inhabited by hundreds of monkeys. When I visited with friends a few years earlier, I was warned not to ask for a child from the temple as it is believed that children requested from this site will have the active and mischievous characteristics of a monkey. Children requested from other shrines such as Jao Phor Seua or Luang Phor Sathorn are said to be difficult to raise as you cannot scold them, for they remain children of the deities, and may return to them if the deities are offended in some way. For this reason some informants like Naa were too scared to ask:

> On one hand I wanted to go, on the other hand I thought, 'Oh people say if you go to ask the Gods for a baby they will be hard to raise. If I raise the child then the Gods might want to take it back.' So I thought about that as well. If you believe in asking for a child then you also have to believe what people say about it.... I had a lot of people tell me: 'Go here! Go there!' But after the miscarriage I went and only asked if I would have another baby ... [but] to ask for a baby from the Gods, I wasn't brave enough, I was scared. I was afraid that I wouldn't look after the baby in the right way. It isn't that I don't believe in it. I'm scared so I'd better not. Because I mightn't do it properly.

Likewise, Porn and Aruth had visited shrines to make merit but had not asked specifically for a child: 'People around us say go and ask! But my mum said "Don't!" She is scared that if we go and ask and receive it [the baby] will be difficult to raise and so I am not brave enough and never ask.' Instead of asking in person, Porn's mother-in-law asks on their behalf.

Conclusions: Enchantment and the Management of Unpredictability

Throughout the world, people employ a variety of culturally specific strategies to ensure their health and manage uncertainty and risk.

The sites and pilgrimages described by the participants in this study highlight the continuation of religious influences in the fashioning of everyday life and health in Thailand and the desire of patients to be proactive amidst the uncertainties of their treatment. It allows them a means of intervening in the unpredictable vagaries of conception.

The diversity of sites visited by infertile couples demonstrates the small spiritual acts and enchantment of everyday life common to the management of health, risks and concerns in Thailand (Nilsen 2011: 1625). It highlights the intermingling of religion and magic and the pluralistic resources commonly utilized by Thais. The circuits through this sacred geography by individuals may differ depending upon the particular request, ethnic or regional allegiances or personal history or preferences. Regarding infertility, these circuits are also gendered. Undertaken predominantly by women, they often involve female deities and figures with no male intermediaries – a source of female agency among women who are disempowered through their infertility. Direct appeals to deities at shrines may also be read as a resort to alternate powers outside of authorized Buddhism, in particular for women in that it does not require male intermediaries such as monks.

The pilgrimages described in this chapter carry a set of common elements. Whether Buddha images, guardian spirits, Chinese deities or Royal spirits, they all involve complementary processes of accessing potent *saksit* powers. Worshipful respect (*bucha*) is demonstrated to all these sources of sacred power through obeisance (*wai phra*) and reverence for objects and personages. As therapeutic places, these shrines are assigned sanctity through association with history, miracles and legends. Some carry particular ethnoregional significance, such as Ya Mo, or Phra That Phanom for northeasterners, or Doi Suthep for northerners, but all are accessible regardless of ethnicity or region. Importantly, most do not require intervention through orthodox institutions but are directly accessible to individuals.

Requests to gods and spirits are enmeshed in the expanding flows of pilgrim-tourists, money, images and merit seeking in Thailand and across the region (Askew 2008; Cohen 1992). They form part of what Pattana Kitiarsa has termed the 'occult economy' of Thailand. As he describes (2007: 133), 'money becomes a form of ritual investment and a means of exchange for religious consumption', whether through the small purchases of flowers and incense, donations to orphanages, larger investments of dance performances, the costs of tours to specific sites, or to purchase food at nearby markets.

Such exchanges are not viewed as mere consumption and commodification, however, but are inherent to the systems of gift exchange and negotiations with the gods. As infertile people, my informants in this study enter into this economy with specific purpose, hence the circuit of sacred sites; 'the sacred geography of fertility' they describe is one among many other itineraries. Multiple circuits overlap depending upon the quest of supplicants: for profit or success in business, for protection from accidents, to cure a disease.

As will be seen in following chapters, in many ways the pilgrimages to shrines by infertile couples find their parallels in the ways in which supplicants also approach the technologies of assisted reproduction. Economic investments in assisted reproductive technologies are significant, but expressed in a language that transmutes cost and commodification into care and investment. Both require faith and trust in a higher authority, as patients follow their faith in the technology and doctors' abilities and reputation. The analogy runs further: the outcome of technological processes of assisted reproduction are doubtful and by no means assured and often seem to hinge upon factors other than mere hormone protocols or the age of the patient. In short, as the doctors themselves wryly note, it is not an exact science (see also Roberts 2006 for a description of Ecuadorian IVF clinics). As they undergo IVF treatment the chances of failure outweigh the chances of success and hence many talk about the role of luck and destiny in their treatment. As I will describe later in this book, patients undergo a range of ritual behaviours in their IVF treatment, especially special diets and bodily disciplines following embryo transfer, and themselves carry a number of beliefs about what one should do to ensure success. Patients use similar language to describe undergoing IVF treatment as a parallel pilgrimage, the self-sacrifice involved in IVF treatment, the purity of their motive and the hope placed upon these interventions. The outcomes of processes like IVF appear magical; there is good reason that the babies that result are described as 'miracle' babies.

In an essay on the production and aesthetics of art, Alfred Gell suggests, 'The enchantment of technology is the power that technical processes have of casting a spell over us so that we see the real world in an enchanted form … the enchantment which is immanent in all kinds of technical activity' (1993: 44). The high-tech production of embryos and babies is full of enchantment, not fully comprehensible to patients participating in it and surprising even the doctors applying it. The enchantment follows from the labyrinthine technical processes, special language and multiple attempts to cater for the individual patient's biology. This casts a magical element over the treatments, whereby seemingly endless faith in the technology and hope is encouraged in even the most difficult cases. The manipulations of the supernatural through visits to shrines or visits to the clinic are not antithetical to the high-tech undertakings of IVF treatment, but follow a continuum of action to produce a 'miracle' child.

Notes

1. Nine is a particularly auspicious number and a similar pilgrimage to nine temples in Bangkok around the Thai new year is a popular activity. The tour she described to Suphanburi is advertised by a number of companies as a day trip and involves cruising along the river to Wat Chalermprakiet Wora Vihan, Wat Kae Nok, Wat Choeng Ta,Wat Choeng Lane, Wat Saeng Siri Dham (for the famous statue of Luang Phor Yim), Wat Yai Sawang Arom,Wat Poramai Yikawas, Wat Sao Tong Thong, Ma Fueng Pagoda (Cambodia Pagoda containing the Ta-Klen Goddess and two statues of topknot child [Kumarn Phom Juk]) and the final temple Wat Phai Lorm to see Phra That Raman Pagoda.
2. This was most notable during the 2007 crisis with King Bhumibol's health (Rama IX) when he was admitted to Siriraj Hospital. Tens of thousands of well wishers crowded Siriraj hospital, many camping in the hospital during his stay, wearing yellow shirts in his honour. The statue of Prince Mahidol was a focus of devotional acts during this time.

Chapter 4

Engaging Technologies

How could we be capable of disenchanting the world, when every day our laboratories and our factories populate the world with hundreds of hybrids stranger than those of the day before? – Latour, *We Have Never Been Modern*, 115

In the previous chapter I described the sacred geography of fertility across Thailand. Infertility clinics form part of that landscape, visited by couples with similar feelings of faith and hope – they offer opportunities for mediation of conception through mysterious and seemingly miraculous medical technologies. In this chapter I consider further the enchantment offered within clinics; as couples engage with reproductive technologies, they do so with faith and trust in the technologies, meticulously following doctors' advice and repeatedly engaging in a series of embodied interventions, tests and examinations.

Monica Bonaccorso (2009: 75) writes of the 'hyper-medicalization of the infertile couple as the most powerful representational strategy in infertility treatment'. By this she means that as infertility becomes pathologized, more and more complex interventions are justified on the basis of the presence of pathology and new procedures and interventions become 'normalized', particularly if procedures fail. 'If the couple is *ill*, clinicians can continually establish reasons for undergoing treatment – particularly when the programme fails.'

I also suggest that the technical activities of IVF themselves, the monitoring, ritualized protocols and interventions upon the body cast their own forms of enchantment over the patients and clinicians (Gell 1992). Both patients and doctors require acts of faith and belief in the efficacy of the technologies. Although the high technology of assisted reproduction is sought out to enable couples to become pregnant, it is also perceived as subject to an element of chance, destiny or karma at work in determining who successfully produces a take-home baby. The experience of repeated failed cycles do not necessarily damage the general faith placed in the technologies; rather, the bodies and actions of the couple, not the technologies, become invested with responsibility for failures. For clinicians the lack of predictable outcomes seems to add to the mystique.

Many people find that the experience of undertaking assisted reproduction itself becomes all-encompassing – or as Sarah Franklin described it, 'a way of life' (1998: 85). Women in particular speak of giving up work to undertake their treatment, finding it both impractical to combine work and commuting with the endless appointments and inconsistent with their vision of future motherhood. But as this chapter illustrates, these visions of a future pregnancy are 'tentative' (Franklin 1997: 135) – the majority of couples undergoing assisted reproduction will not succeed in achieving a take-home baby. This chapter is also about the lived experiences of failure and success in the clinics and how couples negotiate and make decisions about continuing treatment. I describe how couples experience various aspects of treatment, from decisions to undertake assisted reproduction through to the various technical interventions.

Choosing a Doctor

Patients made decisions over where to undertake assisted reproductive treatment based upon a constellation of factors such as reputation of the doctor, hospital or clinic reputation and price. Some had discussed various clinics with other doctors, but most self-referred. Proximity was an important consideration for some patients, but others were prepared to travel several hours and deal with Bangkok's congested traffic to seek services with a particular doctor. Word of mouth was particularly important, with many couples stating that they choose a particular doctor or clinic because friends at work had recommended them or had success with that doctor. For people based in Bangkok there are numerous choices. For example, Mot noted: 'There were so many places for us to choose such as R Private Hospital and P Private Hospital but we weren't sure about their doctors. Moreover, about three people from work had succeeded with this doctor so we were confident [to come here to the public clinic].'

For some patients, the costs determined where they sought treatment. Undertaking IVF is expensive and beyond the reach of the lower classes. Even for middle class Thais the costs involve considerable sacrifice. Kwan went to one private clinic only to find the costs daunting. To save costs she underwent the cheaper treatment of IUI but without success and was now undergoing IVF:

> Y (private) clinic is expensive so I went there to have the test and was about to start the first stage. But the cost of the test was really expensive, for an examination only it cost 7,000 baht. It was only a blood test, not even an internal examination. So when they made an appointment for the results I didn't turn up and just called for the results and then I went for treatment at X (public) hospital instead for about two years and had IUI three times.

As the Thai national health policy and private health insurance makes no provisions to cover infertility treatment, the cost of treatment is borne by infertile couples out of pocket. The difference between public and private treatment therefore lies in costs from an average US $2,900 per cycle in government hospitals to US $5,800 or more per cycle in private centres (Vutyavanich et al. 2011). Even within public hospitals assisted reproductive technologies are only accessible to the middle and upper classes. Hence for patients such as Kwan with limited resources, there was little choice but to pursue treatment in the public system. Likewise, Ladda was shocked at the costs of treatment:

> Before the third attempt, I saw another patient was paying for her bills. She was complaining that she'd spent her second million already and still was not sure if it would work for her. I was shocked to hear that because I did not have a lot of money then. I just wanted to have a baby. Where would I get the money from? Let alone worrying about the second million, I did not even have the first million!

Wealthier patients have more choice but many of them also choose to attend clinics of the public university teaching hospitals such as Siriraj and Chulalongkorn because of the prestige and reputation of these hospitals as the leading medical institutions of Thailand. As several noted, even His Majesty the King of Thailand attends Siriraj Hospital.

Many patients emphasized service above reputation and chose smaller private clinics for the more personalized treatment they offered. Nit and Ton emphasized the need for good service:

> We should get the service that we pay for. If you don't get good service that you pay for you feel bad.... Some staff they know their duties and think that patients know it as well. We came here because we were impressed with how they care for us and secondly the travelling (the proximity). If we decided to go to (another private hospital) we'd have to go to see them and struggle with the traffic.... I am impressed with the doctor and all the hospital's staff here, especially the nurses and reception. The most important thing is they respect us and look after us very well.

Ton added: 'No matter how good the doctor is, if nurses and staff were not good, we would not want to come back. Other hospitals still lack this. We could have gone to other big hospitals where we came from but we prefer to come here.'

Beginning Treatment

The stories from patients draw attention to the fact that most are self-referred. It is not common for Thai patients to regularly see a general practitioner who then refers them. Patients typically seek specialist care themselves, either through attending a public gynaecology clinic from which they are then referred or making a private appointment. Ladda described how her first attempt to seek treatment ended in her walking away due to fear:

> I was so nervous and scared. I went to B hospital before I went to the R Hospital. I was in a waiting room. As soon as my name was called out, I was so embarrassed and walked out to the car park. My husband did not understand why I waited for three hours and then threw it all away. We had to wait for that doctor for a long time ... not that there were many patients but the doctor did not arrive on time.

Standard clinical protocols for infertile couples usually involve some initial history taking and attempting to fall pregnant naturally using the ovulation method, followed by some testing and IUI with hormonal treatment to enhance ovulation. If this is not successful after several cycles, couples usually undergo further investigations and interventions, all of which can take many months or even years. Eventually when lower-tech alternatives have been exhausted, a couple may be considered candidates for in vitro fertilization.

For example, Nari is thirty-seven years old; her husband is forty-three and they own their own business in Bangkok. She and her husband discovered they were infertile in their sixth year of marriage after they failed to become pregnant two years after discontinuing contraception. They consulted a specialist who put Nari on fertility drugs. 'At the first hospital, the treatment was to count the day that we had sexual relations and take some hormones. We gave up after trying that for about four or five cycles with no success. Then we went to another hospital.' At that hospital they commenced IUI and were fortunate to fall pregnant on their first attempt. 'I was quite nervous on the first time [with IUI] because I never even had any internal examination before. I had to be OK with it because I really wanted to have a child. I felt weird at first, especially when I thought of my husband helping himself to collect his semen.'

She was around thirty-four years old when her first child was born. Now that her daughter is over two years old they are now trying for a second child. So far they have tried IUI again five times without success. They are now on their second cycle of IVF: 'I thought the second time would be as easy as the first time. My expectation might have been too high.'

Some patients expressed dissatisfaction with the low-tech interventions such as IUI and said they were relieved when their doctor allowed them to commence IVF as they believed it would increase their chances of success. Kwan had undergone treatment at another hospital:

> When it [a pregnancy] didn't stick we stopped and moved here to do a test tube baby. The doctor got our history and I told him the story.... He accepted that our history was like this and listened to us about when we did IUI what it was like and so he checked again and then started a test tube baby.... He gives us confidence he doesn't want us to spend a lot of money, not have a lot of pain, but we are impatient. Really he would like us to do IUI one more time but I told him altogether it would be five times so we don't want it. Five times is five months, it wastes time. So I asked to start doing a test tube baby and he accepted that.

Low-tech interventions are described as a waste of time for women whose chances of a successful pregnancy decrease as they age. Ploy likewise spoke of her age and not having time to pursue low-tech technologies. She describes IVF as 'the ultimate' option: 'The doctor told me that I could still try the injection but not more than three times. I am thinking that I am not young anymore. I have to wait every time I come for the injection and cannot do anything much.

I think that the IVF is the ultimate option, and then I can come to terms with it if I still cannot be pregnant this way. I would be able to put all of my energy to my work or something else.'

The cost of IVF can be a barrier. Although eager to try, Ploy had to consider carefully her financial situation. She consulted friends before deciding to go ahead with treatment.

> I talked to a friend of mine who had the IVF experience before. Her ovary did not respond with the medication very well. She only got three embryos and could not use all three at once, so she had to start over from the beginning process again. She said that she still wanted to do it again but she needed more time to prepare herself. She has no problem with money. On the other hand, another close friend of mine, who knows more about my financial situation, did not understand why I want to have a baby so badly. I had to reconsider, after I spoke with her, that I could not compare myself with the other friend. Then, I called another friend, who is in the same kind of job [and in a similar financial situation] to get her opinion about having kids. I wanted to know if it was really hard and expensive. She did not seem to think that there were problems so I felt better and decided to go ahead [with the treatment].

Practices of Visualization

Treatment for infertility involves a continuous process of scrutiny, visualization and medical monitoring. Throughout the procedures undertaken within infertility clinics, a range of scientific practices are used for seeing and knowing about body parts, gametes and embryos. These include a range of visualization techniques such as laparoscopic technologies, the use of dyes to investigate fallopian tubes, microscopic counts of sperms and confirmation of embryo development, to ultrasounds and three-dimensional ultrasounds of pregnancies. Doctors often take videos of surgical procedures which are later given to patients as evidence of what has been done during surgery. Transvaginal ultrasounds are taken to confirm ovulation and predict the number of eggs prior to collection. If pregnant, ultrasounds are used to check development and reassure parents-to-be of the normality of the foetus.

Procedures such as vaginal examinations, transvaginal ultrasounds and artificial insemination cause embarrassment and discomfort for women. Porn described her acute shame at having a male doctor insert the transvaginal ultrasound device, explaining that: 'In Thai culture, if it is not our husband we don't want to reveal ... something like that [the vagina]. ... If it is a female nurse then it doesn't matter, a little bit embarrassing but less. The same with IUI, it is a man who did the IUI injection. I believe every woman wouldn't feel comfortable especially ... with someone you only see once!'

Public display of private parts of the body underscores the fact that within the clinic the act of conception is removed from the intimate spaces of a couples' relationship into the public biomedical gaze. As women become socialized into the hypermedicalized world of IVF, such feelings of embarrassment, so acutely felt at first, become distanced as they become positioned as collaborating observers of their body processes. As a woman adopts the medicalized, pathologized view of her body, she undergoes a gradual transformation into a collaborator viewing their bodies as raw lab material for reproduction.

Measurement technologies are also used extensively, so ova and individual spermatozoa are measured as evidence of whether they are viable or unviable, sperm counts are undertaken, the thickness of the endometrial lining of a woman's uterus is measured. Patients become socialized into such views of their bodies, seeing the hidden depths of their reproductive systems and reading strange shadows and bumps as evidence of bodily disorder and anomaly. They become skilled at citing their numbers of eggs, thickness of linings, the sizes of heads of sperm. Videos, scans and ultrasound pictures are often kept as memorabilia, either for future reference by other clinicians, or for the child-to-be as evidence of the efforts of their parents. The medical monitoring finds its parallel in monitoring by family and friends. Many women described repeated questions from in-laws in particular, about their treatment and pregnancy status, that some found far from helpful. The self-monitoring by women can be intense. Mot (thirty-four years old) for example, described how during her use of IUI and later IVF she became fixated upon pregnancy testing:

> I bought so many pregnancy tests. I knew that my period was due every third of each month. I already used the test since on the first. My husband had to stop me because I just wanted to keep testing it on the second, third, fifth and the sixth day until the period came. I cried after losing hopes so many times. It messed with your head a lot. My husband had to make a rule for me to do the test only once and I had to wait for a week before I could do it so that I would not be so sad. This time, I did not realize that I was pregnant until the ninth or the tenth day. I did not realize that I did not have a period and did not do the test until a work colleague asked me how I went with the doctor.

> The work colleague bought the pregnancy test from a 7-Eleven store for me. I let my husband know once we'd found out about the pregnancy. He was openly, extremely excited. He asked to see the result if it was really real. He told his mother and his mother told everyone else. They were so happy.

Within such visual and technical vocabulary of the clinics, 'success' can be defined in many ways. Although ultimately 'success' is defined as a live birth to a healthy child and mother, 'success' talk is used throughout the process of IVF: to define good ovarian response to hormonal stimulation, the collection of a sufficient number of 'beautiful' ova, the discovery of even a few viable sperm, the achievement of correct thickness of endometrium. It is noticeable how often women and men undergoing treatment can cite these technical mantras, albeit sometimes incorrectly, as evidence of successful response of their bodies. An embryonic implantation is defined as a 'pregnancy' and included in pregnancy outcome figures of clinics even though the majority of these will miscarry. These successes encourage the patient to feel their bodies are achieving normality, or even overachieving, despite their infertile status. Success talk is used to encourage them to continue their attempts in further cycles.

Enmeshed in the Process

Franklin (1998: 107) described the ways in which women in Britain feel obliged to utilize the range of technological interventions available: 'Although ARTs are often celebrated as an expansion of reproductive choice, all the women interviewed for this study described not having any choice – they "had to try" IVF.' She describes the ways in which technological developments construct the boundaries of choice and desire for particular treatment. This becomes an all-consuming aspect of patient's lives in terms of their money, time, emotions, pain and relationships. They are aware of the difficulties of undergoing ARTs. Women in her study 'expressed two primary aims in relation to IVF: if they succeeded, they would achieve the ultimate goal of a take-home baby, and if they failed, at least they would know that they had tried everything. This pair of alternate resolutions was seen to *guarantee success* – one way or another, a positive outcome was assured' (emphasis in original).

As new treatment options become available to women and they feel closer to a pregnancy than ever before, many find it difficult to step away from the desire and promise held with trying one more cycle. Becker (2000: 116) describes assisted reproductive technologies as 'selling hope'. She describes how couples become 'enmeshed, and then entrapped, in the process' (2000: 165), submitting to increasingly more complex interventions (see also Franklin 1997).

In this book, couples interviewed related remarkably similar sentiments – trying IVF to reassure themselves and others they had done all they could to try to have a child. For example, after trying IUI five times with no success Porn and Aruth decided to undertake IVF:

> So we did IUI for five times without any success so the doctor said well then IVF. So we talked to each other as to whether we were going to do this or not as it costs a lot of money. And my husband said 'Let's just go for it' [*hai man sud sud pay loei*]. If we don't do it now and later want to do it at least we we'll know that we have done our best. [If] we don't have it, we don't have it. So we decided to do it.

Repeated attempts at using assisted reproduction are rhetorically framed within positive language of persistence, resolve (thanjai), struggling (su) and trying one's best (พยายามเต็มที่). As Nari stated: 'We think that we gave our best for the baby to become our child.' The sense of 'trying one's best' is common within IVF narratives (Franklin 1997: 173–175) in the sense that knowing that one has tried will assuage any future regrets and give couples peace of mind. As will be discussed further in chapter 6 it also demonstrates a determination to fulfil 'normative' gender expectations, especially for women.

Only one of the clinics in which I worked offered dedicated nurse-counsellors to support patients (see chapter 5). As a result most patients are reliant upon their appointments with their doctors for information and support. For many patients, especially those within the public hospitals, the heavy caseloads and limited time for appointments means they are able to receive only limited counselling. None of the clinics in which I worked had any patient support groups or forums in which patients could get to know one another. Some public clinics offer regular weekend public information sessions for people wishing to understand the process and options for infertility treatment. For example, Chulalongkorn offers a monthly information session which is very popular. For the most part there are only limited interactions between patients at clinics. As I will discuss in chapter 7, the Internet has become a popular means for people to receive information and social support.

Most women undergoing treatment reported receiving most support from their partners and close family members. For example, Pui said her husband, siblings, sisters and family members say 'All the best! I wish you success! Keep trying!' and in some cases parents helped pay for treatment. In some cases couples had kept their treatment secretive and not told family members and so had no avenues for support other than themselves. Kwan stated that her parents and siblings on both side gave her and her husband the most support during treatment, although this can also be a form of familial surveillance adding further pressure: 'They constantly ask. And when I say I have a period they are disappointed. They wait anxiously to see if I have a period or not, and when I say I have they feel disappointed.'

Hormones

A range of hormonal medications are used in assisted reproduction. Typically a woman will have been prescribed medications to enhance her fertility while trying to conceive naturally or with the use of IUI. If she undergoes an IVF cycle, her menstrual cycle will be stopped by hormones and restarted using drugs to stimulate ova production and ovulation for collection, often involving daily abdominal injections and in some cases nasal administration. Some women may also be given further drugs to induce production of their endometrium. Finally, should implantation take place and show signs of a threatened miscarriage, women may be given further hormonal treatment to support the pregnancy. The management of the administration and timing of these drugs was a frequent cause of concern and frustration for many women interviewed. For those who lived far from their clinic, arrangements had to be made for the administration of the daily injections, either involving daily trips to the clinic in heavy traffic or finding a nearby practitioner to assist. Only two couples reported self-administering the injections. Sometimes patients found they had miscalculated the amount of medication needed and had to return to the clinic to purchase more. If the timing of ovulation was missed, ova could not be collected and their effort on that cycle would be lost and the process repeated all over again.

Few women complained about side effects and only did so in response to direct probes. Those that did tended to comment about physical effects: dizziness, bloating, nausea and breast tenderness and the pain of injections. Kwan, for example, said: 'I have had no emotional changes, I'm normal but feel that my weight has increased, like I am bloated, because it is a hormone, it is strong. I'm very buxom also, only this. No mood changes.' Mot was one of the few women to report emotional responses to treatment: 'It was not a very nice time then. After the operation, I had to take some medications to stop the period. During that time, I had symptoms like having menopause. I was so irritable, temperamental, had hot flashes and sweaty. I had those symptoms for over three months and was so unapproachable. My husband was wary of me.' Porn described a variety of effects from the hormones she used:

> We have stimulants in tablet forms and also hormones and some that is a nasal spray lots of things. But all must be hormones. There is one I used that started to give me a moustache and facial hair. I had mood swings. There was a time at which no matter what you said it wouldn't be right. I had never felt like this before, I wasn't sure if it was due to the hormones or not but I think it is.

Ying noted her body has been affected by the drugs used but then contradicted this with her observation that it was 'natural' (*thammachaat*) and hence not a concern:

> During the period of treatment my siblings said, 'Don't do it! It may affect your body.' It is true it has wrecked it. Pregnant woman are fat and stimulants make you fat. When I started I weighed 45 kilos and I got as fat as 63 kilos, it's hard to lose weight. Hormones are all through my body now. I used to wear size A bra and now I wear E size. It takes time to reduce.
>
> There shouldn't be a lot of effects as what we have done, we have only done to the womb and so it isn't any different from giving birth because people who give birth don't do anything to other parts of their body, it doesn't affect their arms and legs. The womb is like a balloon. Like those who have a caesarean section, you know, the mothers lie on the surgical table and the doctors cut along a line and even lift the womb up and [all] that is natural.

Ying's description of the drug regimens as simply affecting one part of her body, the womb, reflects the degree to which she has disembodied the process of assisted conception, viewing her body as a collection of parts – a womb, an endometrium – that is a result of the hypermedicalization of reproduction. Disruption of the womb through drugs, surgery or curettage of the endometrium, is described as mimicking 'natural' (*thammachaat*) processes, the womb a mere vessel or expandable balloon to be manipulated. By imitating nature, assisted reproduction thus redefines 'the natural'. And because it is natural, it cannot be harmful. Few women worried about possible long-term side effects for themselves; rather they were understood as transitory. The only mention of long-term effects came from Poy's husband who feared the hormones may 'cause cancer because the stimulants might destroy the womb'.

Heather Paxson (2003) argues that in Greece assisted reproduction is described as working with nature, rather than in opposition to it. Women depict themselves as morally responsible for maintaining or treating their bodies to facilitate the technological making of their babies to overcome their childlessness. We can see this also operating in Ying's statement about the hormones she uses being 'natural'. Her use of the term *thammachaat* highlights how Thai concepts of 'nature' and what is 'natural' can be broader than the concept in the English language. *Thammachaat* is a compound word derived from Sanskrit, *thaama* (dharma) or Buddhist law or truth, and *chaat,* meaning 'life' and in some instances 'nation' (Stott 1991). As a term it may include places and things that are human-made but not disruptive of the dharmic order, hence there is not a strict opposition between that natural and 'human-made'. Such a usage can be seen in this example by Ying where she declares that the hormones she uses are as natural as those normally circulating in the body during pregnancy. They do not disrupt the normal order of things. But such a usage of *thammachaat* applied to assisted reproduction is unstable. For example, in the situation in the lift described at the beginning of this book, the patient asks another woman if her baby is *thammachaat* – made without the mediation of IVF. Here we are left to consider whether this represents a shifting meaning of *thammachaat* closer to the understandings of 'nature' as used in English, or if she is implying that a baby conceived without IVF represents dharmic order more truthfully.

Ova Collection

After a period of hormonal stimulation through injections or drugs, ova collection is timed to coincide with the maturity of the ova. The experience of ova collection was described by women as one of anywhere from mild discomfort to severe pain. Women are anxious to know the number and quality of the eggs collected and often see the production of a small number of eggs as a failure. A small number of eggs decreases the chances of a successful fertilization and may require a patient to go through the expensive and painful ova stimulation and collection process again if she wishes to undertake further cycles. On the other hand, an excessive number of eggs may mean they are not of sufficient size and quality for successful fertilization. Pook described her experience of ova collection:

> If you can't come early then you have to stay overnight at the hotel the night before. If you come late the eggs will drop. So we had to come early. Arriving here at 7 AM waiting for the doctor. If the eggs fall everything you have done so far [with the IVF] means nothing. I remember that I didn't sleep deeply and have a feeling that I heard the doctor say 'four eggs'. Very few. When I came for the ultrasound I had twenty-four eggs. I heard the doctor say, 'She has twenty-four eggs.' Where did they go? So I started to fret. Why are there so few? I wanted to ask the doctor exactly how many eggs I got but the doctor left before I could. I asked my friend how many eggs she got and she said over ten and the other patients who had eggs collected on that day got seven to eight. I think I got four eggs. Very few. If I do it and they don't stick then I have to start again and waste more money. Rich people have so many eggs, while people with no money are trying their best and get very few eggs. But I have to ask the doctor again because that is what I heard. I heard everything and I felt the doctor stir something in my vagina. I felt that I would like the doctor to finish the egg collection quickly. It hurt. Seems like the doctor used some kind of equipment. I felt that from when he started doing it [collect the eggs] as I could still feel things. If I have a lot [of eggs] it is good but I have only a few. I asked friends and they said they had a lot, why have I so few eggs?

Gae seems to have had little idea of what ova collection would involve and found the experience confronting:

> First I asked the doctor and he said it would be like an internal examination. [When I got in the op room] it was Oooo! Heck! They had to put me to sleep. When I reached the op room I was terrified.
>
> Interviewer: So the doctor didn't tell you about this before?
>
> Maybe he said I would have to be put to sleep but I didn't know it was to be done in the op room so it was scary, all green and all the measurements and equipment to monitor.... After I changed my dress they take your heart rate and blood pressure and give you anaesthetic. He did tell me before I entered the room he said there would be a machine to suck the eggs out, that it might hurt a little so that they give you anaesthetic. After I woke I felt a bit nauseous and dizzy.
>
> Interviewer: Did it hurt?

> It didn't hurt after I woke but after I returned home about 12 or 1 PM then it started to hurt I think that the painkiller had worn off.

She was pleased that fifteen eggs had been collected:

> At first when I came to stimulate the eggs the doctor said that my ovaries don't ovulate at all. Even though I increased the medication. And I thought, 'Oh! I'm not normal in that way!' So they increased it to two needles a day for many days. Before the last day when they checked before collecting the eggs the doctor said I have five or six eggs. And the other tube didn't have eggs at all. Oooo, it was so few! Not normal? Then when they collected them the doctor said unexpectedly 'fifteen eggs' and I felt oh so happy! And then the nurse called and said the babies' cells are dividing really well. Thirteen [blastocycsts] they all divided. And so I felt better.

Pook reported considerable pain following collection: 'You feel the pain. It hurt a lot. Breast tenderness. The side effect is breast tenderness, stomach ache and I had to take paracetamol against the pain. Just felt better today. Every day I lay down in pain but it was bearable. Not that it is unbearable. I don't know whether other people felt like this, I haven't asked anyone.'

A number of other studies report concern from patients about the possible mixing up of gametes during IVF procedures. These were generally associated with religious concerns about the legitimacy of the child produced and the maintenance of religious purity. For example, Susan Martha Kahn (2000: 113–114) reports that for Orthodox Jewish couples in Israel, extremely strict regulations and protocols, including the presence of ultra-Orthodox women observers or *maschgichot* to supervise lab procedures, ensure there is no inadvertent mixing up of gametes which might result in rabbinically proscribed unions. Likewise, Inhorn (2003a: 117–118) reports that among Sunni and Coptic Christian Egyptian couples with anxiety about possible mistakes in the lab, videotaping of the lab procedures in one clinic offered some reassurance.

In contrast, no Thai patients self-reported anxieties over lab mistakes. This was somewhat surprising given the strong discourse over the importance of 'bloodlines' expressed by many interviewees. When asked, most did not know what the procedures in their clinic were to ensure correct gametes were used, although some had noticed the name labels attached to sperm samples and presumed there was a system in place. They placed great trust in the clinic staff not to tamper with gametes (see chapter 5 for more details).

All clinics had careful labelling procedures and some had protocols ensuring that only one set of gametes was manipulated within the lab at any one time. Some clinics also offered videotaping of the laboratory procedures providing couples with an opportunity to witness the fertilization/injection procedures (even though this in itself does not allow for the clear identity of the gametes used to be confirmed). The embryologist from one private clinic explained their procedures for ensuring that there were no mix-ups of sperm or ova samples and noted that if a couple was particularly concerned they might be offered to physically witness the lab work:

> We need to identify each patient in each single step from start to the end of procedures. Let's say one patient arrives at the counter, a nurse will get his name and write down on the sperm container. Then the patient will collect his sperms and bring the container back himself. During the procedures that involve a courier, the courier will have to have a request form and a specimen form from the patient. Both a nurse and a courier need to sign on the delivery and pick-up time. A nurse has to confirm the request form – if it has the right name on it. At the lab, we will work on one at the time. We will not line them up and then work on them. Then we will type the patient's name on a sticker to prevent misspelling. Once the sperms get to the doctor, he will check the patient's name and surname and call out the name before injecting them back.

She noted that some of their 'well-educated' patients ask how they know that the embryos are theirs: 'We sometimes take a picture of the embryos and they are still unsure so we have to explain about the procedures to them. And if that does not help, we will get them to observe the procedures themselves.'

Transfer

After incubation, the petri plates are examined to see how well the cells are dividing. At this point they are screened, some are defined by laboratory staff as *suay*, 'beautiful', others that are not dividing well will be discarded. At this point many private clinics will phone the patient to tell them about the development. The 'beautiful' blastocysts will then be transferred to the woman or surrogate's womb and then a period of waiting takes place to see if the pregnancy 'sticks', or implants, and continues to develop normally. The period around transfer is the most stressful for women. It is a time of excitement at the prospect of a successful pregnancy, but also of enormous stress due to the knowledge that most pregnancies were not successful. Women described themselves as being 'pregnant' and feeling special with the knowledge that a life was inside them.

Ritualized behaviours surround embryo transfer. Becker (2000: 162–163) notes in her study the sense of ceremony surrounding transfer – a sense of mystery established through a special quiet dark room, the liminal state of the woman patient who is placed in an awkward physical position face down with her bottom exposed and elevated, a sense of suspense as the live embryos are injected via a catheter, only whispering allowed following the transfer while the women rests. It is a transformative ritual turning her into a pregnant mother, if only for a short time. Likewise in the Thai clinics I studied, women described a range of ritualized acts surrounding transfer. Patients arrive early for the transfer which takes place in a surgical room, which in some clinics is darkened and warm. Partners were not present during the transfer but waited outside until the women emerged following a period of incumbent rest. Private patients received photographs of their embryos, humanized even before they are inserted into a woman's body. Women describe the thrill of knowing they had live embryos inside them. Transformed by the process, women then face a period of waiting to find out if the pregnancy will 'stick'. Pui complained that she felt she was not given enough information on what she should do after the transfer: 'They simply say don't use stairs, don't ride the bike. That's all they say and "Don't lift heavy stuff". But they don't explain in detail what I should do.' The process of implantation is viewed as a delicate process, in which the slightest bump or abdominal push will disrupt the process and result in a miscarriage. This harks back to early Thai understandings of early pregnancy in traditional medical texts such as the *Thai Book of Genesis* (*Khampee prathom chinda*):

> At the time of conception they say that [the embryo] is the finest particle, so fine ... having been conceived in the mother's womb it can become liquefied more than seven times a day, it is so difficult to retain.... When the pregnancy has lasted seven days without miscarriage the blood becomes thicker, like water which has been used to wash meat. After another seven days it becomes flesh. (Mulholland 1989: 17)

Many women imposed a period of rest upon themselves following embryo transfer, some lying down in bed in self-imposed confinement for two weeks or more following transfer and taking great care with bowel movements so as not to push with the abdominal muscles (see, for example, Nut in chapter 6). Manit explained: 'For those who have IVF, it's not natural conception. To walk, to move, or whatever, it has to be like creeping, slow motion.' Following her embryo transfer, Ladda explained:

> I stopped everything. I acted like a moron. I did not even carry my bag. I refused to go upstairs and slept right here [downstairs] and being gentle with everything. I did not even lift my finger and hired a maid to do things for me. I heard that a friend of my friend had problems with her pregnancies. She had miscarriages about three or four times and had to stay still under a drip so she could finally be pregnant. I just assumed that it was something I had to do.... The doctor did not say anything about it. He did not want us to be so worried about it but I heard from other patients that I should not move, should not urinate too hard because I might lose the embryos along with the urine. It's like a myth that people believe. I did not tell the doctor about this because I felt embarrassed that I did more than what the doctor told me to do.

Others reported avoiding certain foods following transfer, according to humoral principles followed by pregnant women. Humorally hot foods are believed to cause a pushing wind which could upset the humoral balance of the women's body leading to a miscarriage. Hence foods such as pickled foods, alcohol or durian are avoided. Such understandings of implantation also lead women to blame themselves and feel guilty when implantation does not occur. Women question whether cycles failed due to their actions or failure to take sufficient care.

There is no medical evidence that such extreme care improves the chances of successful implantation, yet many women suggested that such behaviour was prudent. According to Poy: 'The doctor said, "Just do things normally." According to the pamphlet [given by the hospital] you can just do what you normally do but I feel it should be extra careful. I must walk carefully and should rest because the last two times it wasn't successful because I walked around to teach and didn't take enough care so this time I will be more careful.'

Phet likewise was going to stay in Bangkok following her third attempt at embryo transfer instead of travelling four hours back home: 'I was so hopeful but it did not work (sigh). One of my husband's cousins had the treatment but not here. They are now having twins but they said they stayed in a hotel right after the implantation process.'

Masae Kato and Margaret Sleeboom-Faulkner (2011) describe how in Japan the period after transfer is a time of 'psuedo-pregnancy' during which prospective parents feel a sense of responsibility for the healthy condition of the foetus and tend to blame themselves for its underdevelopment or failure. In Thailand there is a social expectation that women should be mindful during pregnancy, avoiding anything that may affect the health or disposition of the unborn child. This extends to attempts to avoid unpleasant sights, sounds, smells and emotions, all of which are said to disturb the child within and can affect the child's development and character. Pregnant women generally pay close attention to their diets, not only nutritionally but by avoiding foods considered 'taboo' during pregnancy, such as 'hot' foods which may affect the humoral balance of their body, causing premature labour winds to flow through their body. All of these precautions seem heightened for women in pregnancy after utilizing assisted technologies.

In some respects the period of seclusion and rest following transfer finds its equivalent in Thai postpartum practices of secluded rest while women 'stay by the fire'. Postpartum 'mother roasting' involves a period during which a woman lies on a special bed near a small fire to warm her body to balance her cold humoral state following birth from five to eleven days (Whittaker 2002a). It is understood as a prophylactic health practice to ensure the health and continued fertility of a woman's womb, realign her body and ensure the production of plentiful breast milk. Symbolically the period of seclusion also marks her transition into full adult status as a mother/nurturer (Keyes 1984; Kirsch 1985; Muecke 1984). Both rituals involve dietary regimes, restricted mobility within a domestic space, no normal work duties, sexual abstinence and physical denial. The secluded rest following transfer is both understood as helping implantation, but also marks a symbolic transition of a woman into a mother, undergoing physical sacrifice while she nurtures the life in her womb.

Multiple Transfers

The practice of transferring a single embryo rather than multiple embryos is are being encouraged whenever feasible due to the dangers of higher-order multiple pregnancies for both mothers and babies (Practice Committee of the American Society for Reproductive Medicine 2012). In all my interviews with doctors within the clinics, I asked them all how many embryos they transferred. Without exception, all stated their clinic transferred only two embryos, to avoid complications associated with multiple births. However, in my interviews I came across a number of instances of such protocols being broken. Pressure is sometimes placed upon doctors to transfer numerous embryos in the hope that one or two will implant successfully. Rather than fear the complications and risks of multiple births, the possibility of twins or higher-order multiples was seen as a boon by couples. For example, Nit and Ton explained that they had five embryos transferred.

> We got seven eggs but there were five healthy ones after the insemination. Three [of the five] were in really good condition but the doctor wanted to implant four embryos. We could not freeze only one embryo so we decided to use all five. We decided it would not be worth spending money to freeze one embryo and transfer four. We were so excited at the thought of getting triplets but we have twins. ... After the blood test, I also worried that it would be triplets. Once the doctor told us that it was twins, we were so happy because we have such a little chance to come back and go through the treatment again. We would have to worry about the expenses while we are bringing up a baby. Besides, we would have to wait until the first baby has grown up before we could come back, and we would be too old by then. It's so good to have twins, now, we are happy.

Naa had many embryos transferred because the laboratory informed the doctor that they were not likely to implant: 'The first time we had seven embryos transplanted because they are not strong. The lab said to put in seven because they were not strong. At first I didn't know I thought there were only four.' Despite her small stature, Nuchnari pressured her doctor to transfer three embryos:

> We had five eggs after the selection process. We use three eggs and kept the other two. We were quite nervous of what to do if we got triplets. The doctor did not say anything when my wife told him that she wanted all three. At the ultrasound, the doctor was quite relieved that he found only two eggs. He worried that the mother is tiny so it could lead to premature birth and the rate of surviving is low. He would not worry so much if she was a big girl.

These stories reveal that despite clinicians understanding the risks of multiple births to both the mother and children, they are prepared to break their own protocols under pressure from patients. This suggests the relationship between patient and doctor is complex, with the doctor at times being the expert to whom patients defer, but at other times positioned as service providers deferring to the desires of their client/consumer.

Failure

The statistics reveal a little of the difficulties and loss experienced by patients undergoing treatment. Various procedures carry different rates of success and high rates of failure, miscarriage and ectopic pregnancies. A study of the causes and results of treatment of infertilty couples at Thammasat Hospital between 1999 and 2004 (Chiamchanya and Su-Angkawatin 2008) found that, the pregnancy rate from IUI was reported as 14.8 per cent while those of IVF 32.3 per cent, ICSI 28 per cent and ICSI-PESA (percutaneous epididymal sperm aspiration) 35.3 per cent. The live birth success of these pregnancies is lower, with the Thammasat review showing 19.4 per cent abortion and 6 per cent ectopic pregnancy rates for IUI, 40 per cent abortion and 10 per cent ectopic pregnancy rates for IVF, a 13 per cent abortion rate for ICSI pregnancies and 16.7 per cent abortion rates for ICSI-PESA.

Fifteen days after transfer, women will undertake a blood test to see if their hormone levels indicate a pregnancy. However, often the pregnancy does not implant correctly or fails for another reason. The waiting period until the test is highly stressful for women, and even then the results of the test may be ambiguous, indicating what is termed a 'chemical pregnancy' rather than actual implantation. Women and men commonly described such pregnancies as ones that 'didn't stick', or had trouble 'holding on'.

Pui explained: 'I'm scared [about the blood test] because the first time [last month] it didn't stick and the Dr did it again for me and so I'm waiting for the result. I don't know it yet I would like it to stick because it hurts my body and wastes money.'

Gae felt responsible for her first unsuccessful transfer of three embryos for which she had high hopes after having produced fifteen 'beautiful' eggs. She said her doctor had been certain they would have success: 'After the implantation, he said to us "Don't let me down".' On a follow-up interview with Gae she revealed that her next attempt had also been unsuccessful:

> Everything was fine the first week but it disappeared the week after. The doctor said that it might be because the lining of the uterus was not thick enough for the embryos to hold on to. Both my husband and I were very upset. We could not sleep after we heard the news from the doctor. I was very sad, could not sleep for three nights. Everything was ready and the technology should have helped. It might be my destiny (ดวง) that we cannot be pregnant. I had a lot on my mind.

Ut and Khiat described their distress at two unsuccessful cycles:

> On the first time, we called the hospital after noticing brown blood discharged from my vagina. I was so stressed and cried, wondered why this happened. The discharge, looked like a period, came out even more so we came to the hospital. After found out that my hormone level did not elevate, I felt so sad and cried. I did not know what to do. I tried to be positive and thought that we still have the second chance, but after we were staying in the hospital for four nights on the second round and not succeeded, we started to feel dejected. On the third round, we prepared ourselves for a disappointment. We did not expect much. If it happens, it happens ... just finish the last lot [of ova]. We did not have as high an expectation as on the first round.

Naa experienced a miscarriage on her first cycle:

> The first time I miscarried, I couldn't accept it, I was very, very sad because I had hoped. People said you are only confident when you see the baby delivered safely. But for me even just getting pregnant, we were happy, we weren't prepared for what could happen. I looked after myself and the miscarriage was a shock for many days. My husband gave me support, 'It doesn't matter, we can still try again. Prepare your body to make it ready and we'll try again. It's OK, It's OK. The baby isn't ready to stay with us.' ... I wanted to know. I wanted to know why? Why after it had implanted did I miscarry? The problem came from what? From me? Or from the embryo? During that time I was very confused, I really wanted to know the details. People brought the information but it wasn't enough for me.... The doctor gave some counselling as well. He didn't say much apart from, 'Hmmm. It's because the chromosome of the child wasn't strong enough. It's like he's not complete, he's not strong enough and so didn't implant.'

Naa highlights the ambiguity and limitations inherent in the technological understanding of the process of conception. Despite sophisticated technologies, monitoring, quantities of medical data and the confidence of her clinician, the exact reasons for the failure of this cycle remain unknowable. She questions if 'the problem' was with her or the embryo. No mention is made in her account of the myriad other technological factors such as handling of the embryos, quality of laboratory service or culture medium that may also contribute to failure. The technology remains unquestioned. Her doctor also places blame upon the embryo, using what Monica Bonaccorso calls 'commonplace' language to give a simplified explanation of failure to implant – a weak 'incomplete' (i.e. disabled) embryo without the strength to hold on. Such accessible language of commonplaces replaces medical language to reassure, and suppresses the anxieties, fears and doubts (2009: 67).

Thus though the failure of a cycle could also potentially represent a crisis of belief in the technology, in this case the failings of the embryo and human body are blamed, shifting responsibility. Likewise the cause of the failed cycle is attributed to the mysteries of the supernatural. Her husband's comment that 'the baby isn't ready to stay with us' refers to the belief in Thailand that children remain spirit children until the third day after birth, during which time they may return to the spirit world. Hence miscarriages are often explained through the idea that the spirit child was not yet ready to be reborn but must remain to be reincarnated at the given time according to its fate and karmic cycle. In this way, embryos are attributed will and agency. For example, following a failed attempt at transfer, Nut and Manit commented: 'As I said we intended to take them home but they wouldn't come back with us.' Such findings are similar to those reported in Japan (Kato and Sleeboom-Faulkner 2011: 440) where failed cycles are blamed as a matter of the will power of the embryo itself or due to the parents' imperfection. People utilize these cultural concepts to come to terms with their loss, 'ascrib[ing] powers of decision-making to embryos while at the same time viewing them as their children and questioning their ability to protect them'.

Mai had decided to take a break from IVF after her unsuccessful cycles. Like Naa she sought an explanation for the failed cycle in her own body:

> I don't know what went wrong. I followed the doctor's every advice of what to do. I was not stressed and taking a lot of rest but that still did not work. Perhaps, it was the stress from my high hope, or it might be from the imbalance of my hormones during the ovulation induction.... The second time, we thought it would work because I had a rest for about two months before getting back to the procedures. The doctor did not know why it did not work either. He thought that everything was ready; I had good health, my hormone level and my mental health are fine. Then, the doctor suggested that he might need to look at my uterus with a scope [laparoscopy] to find any abnormality. I wondered why the doctor did not do this from the beginning. The doctor told me that it would be a waste of money because the ultrasound scans should have picked up the abnormalities if there were any. He just did not want us to pay for the extra charges. There was a little bit of fascia that needed to be removed. There was nothing serious, no cysts or anything else. When the doctor asked if I was ready, I said no. I felt that I was not emotionally ready. The first

> trial was not so bad but I felt very disappointed on the second time. We had spent so much money already, and that was not the main problem. The problem was that it put a lot pressure on our emotions and relationship. Sometimes, it led to arguments with no reasons. I was very disappointed with the whole thing so I wanted to take a break for about two months before I came back for the third time.

Her account reveals a common understanding circulating around all clinics, that stress impedes conception. Patients are constantly reminded that stress affects hormonal balance, the production of gametes and implantation. They are advised to relax, not undertake strenuous work and ensure plentiful rest – however difficult this may be amidst the emotional turmoil and physical duress of assisted reproductive treatment. One nurse suggested: 'You can tell which women will fall pregnant just by their stress levels. It always works for the relaxed ones.' For Mai, however, despite her careful preparation stress can also result from 'high hopes'. She admonishes herself for being overly hopeful. She was honest about the strain the failed cycles had placed upon her relationship, causing her to delay a third try. Likewise, Gae promised herself not to hope too much for her next attempt:

> I think a lot when I'm alone. If there are many people around me, I forget and feel a little bit better. It's like something's missing. There were discharges with lumps of blood. I was very sad because it did not look like a normal period. When I came to get the blood test done, the doctor told me that it'd gone, so he did not give me any more suppositories [to prevent miscarriage]. The next day, there were more lumps of blood because of missing the suppository for a day. I feel better now though. I have come to terms with it and I perhaps won't be very sad next time. I thought it would be my luck then because I thought everything was ready, and I was told that the embryos looked great. I won't put too much hope on it next time. If it works, it would be a bonus for me.

There is a sense that each cycle represents a test that a woman should pass – failure is read as 'letting down' the doctor (see Gae's comments above). In this respect doctors sometimes act like coaches or teachers, spurring on their charges with positive words and pep talks. One doctor described his role as helping couples 'maintain hope and a positive attitude'. Nut and Manit likened failure of a cycle to having to repeat a subject of school:

> Nut: He [the doctor] keeps saying all the time that if we fail we have to start it all over again. This made me feel bad.

Manit: It's like you fail exams, you have to study that subject again … the same subject really.

Nut: Compared to, if we fail an exam, we are not going to study again.

Manit: If you fail your exam, you have to start again, same teacher, same subject, same textbook. But if you are more diligent, pay more attention. What is better? [Continuing or giving up.] Right?

A Case Study: Ladda's Story

The case study of Ladda below demonstrates not only the level of physical endurance that epitomizes the experiences of many patients, but how treatment and repeated failures can result in an escalation of increasingly high-tech interventions—from IUI to using donor ova.

Ladda is forty-five years old. She is a small businesswoman who runs two small food stalls at a major shopping centre. Her story reflects both the complexity of the medical history of many patients, as well as her determined persistence to pursue treatment despite multiple setbacks and painful surgery. The interventions upon her body became increasingly complex as she encountered repeated failures. She has been married for twenty-one years and said she has been trying to have a child since she was married. At age thirty, after five years of using no contraception, she went to a general practitioner who gave her IUI, even though he was not a fertility specialist. With no success she did not return for a year. During this time she experienced a serious illness. She lost all her hair, her body swelled and she was experiencing joint pain so she sought help from a number of doctors: 'I went in and out of clinics so often as if I was there for shopping.… I saw so many different doctors but they could not pinpoint what disease exactly.' Finally she went to another hospital where she was then diagnosed as having systemic lupus erythematosus (SLE, an autoimmune disease). But it appears her symptoms may have been iatrogenic:

> They gave me some medications. I had side effects like SLE; my whole body was swollen, I lost all my hair. I had to wear hats or wigs. Initially, I only had problems with no periods and hair lost. I stopped the treatment because for the two months I took the medications, the symptoms got worsen. My face and body were swollen. I gained from thirty-six kilograms to about sixty-six kilograms. I could not get up and had pain in my bones and all around. I was told that steroids caused all these problems. I just stopped the medications and never

> went back to that hospital again. Once I stopped the medications, the symptoms went and I had my hair back again.

Two years later her hair returned and 'the feeling of wanting a child had come back'. As is traditional practice in Thailand, they 'adopted' a four-year-old nephew who came to live and be raised by them. But this has not worked out well:

> It would get worse when his parents came around or called to ask for money. They kept asking the child if he missed them. I think it was like they provoked the child to have problems. The child was crying with them over the phone. It seemed like I was keeping them from each other. It was like I made my nephew call me 'mom'. His mother has gone but his father is still around. The child is very aggressive with us but not with his father. We adopted him when he was four years old, now he is sixteen. He has been with us for twelve years. Adopting a child is not a good thing but I did not know that.... A lot of well-educated people warned me that 'put another man's child in your bosom, and he'll creep out at your elbow'. At the time I thought it was okay because he was my own nephew. I would not mind even if his parents wanted to take him back. I just realize now that whatever those people warned me, it is all true.

Around this time a friend loaned her a book on infertility and IVF by a prominent doctor and this inspired her to attend his clinic to try once again. After a physical examination she was given medication to stimulate the ovary in preparation for IUI. At the ultrasound to find out how many ova had been produced they discovered a cervical tumour. She had immediate surgery to remove the tumour: 'Oh! I'd had so many operations already and spent so much money on the medications. Why didn't you check at the beginning? You've confirmed that everything was OK. I have spent more than ten of thousands baht and now, you just say "sorry" and told me that I had a tumour in my cervix?'

Three months after the surgery her periods returned and she commenced treatment again. Her first and second IUI attempts didn't work. Then on the third attempt she thought it had failed but a blood test revealed her hormones had risen, indicating pregnancy. 'I was so happy. I was already pregnant on the third attempt but I had to be on injections to prevent a miscarriage every second day. I was on the injections for about ten days, the clinic told me that the hormone had gone and it [the pregnancy] was over.'

Following this disappointment she decided to have a break from further treatment. But two years later after a friend's successful infertility treatment she decided to try again at another hospital. But 'destiny intervened' in the form of a regular customer to their phone store who worked at a major public hospital and arranged for Ladda to attend the infertility clinic there. A laproscopic examination revealed a cyst in the right fallopian tube, whereas her left fallopian tube 'was dirty and causing difficulty in getting pregnant but could still be used'. She needed surgery to remove the right tube as it was causing pain, but because of the long waiting list at the public hospital, she had that surgery done at a private hospital. After three months' recuperation she had blood tests to check her hormone levels. The third test revealed she was ready to try again. She took further hormones to stimulate the ovaries this time to undergo an IVF cycle. The first time she produced no ova: 'I had to use the expensive medication.' At the second attempt at ovarian stimulation she only produced three eggs, of which only one was viable. The cycle was unsuccessful:

> After the first round, the doctor told me that I had no hope because no matter how expensive the medication we used, it still could not stimulate the eggs. They were quite straight with me. At the time, I was so upset that I would never have kid. My husband was indifferent; he did not care either way. He felt sorry for me but I was the one who strived to have a baby. I could not bear thinking that I would not have any baby. I could achieve anything ... work wise but why did I lose for this?
>
> Interviewer: Who did you lose to?
>
> Lost to my destiny. I thought that whatever I want, I could always work at it and get it. It was not like I aimed for a star. Nothing was ever impossible for me but why was it so hard for me to have a baby. I already had about four or five operations.

By this time she was around thirty-eight years old. The doctor suggested ova donation: 'He asked how many sisters I had and if it was possible to ask my little sister to help.' Her younger sister, who was then age twenty-five, agreed to act as a donor.

> She has a partner [she is a *mia noi* or mistress] but no children. I told her that I really wanted to have a baby because I did not want to feel that something was missing in my life when I got really old. She agreed that I already had everything in life but the baby, and she wanted my life to be complete. She agreed to do it right away. Though, on that day, I was so afraid that she would say no so I offered her 100,000 baht as well, with the condition that she had to stop working for a month. I think she both wanted the money and

> wanted me to be happy. We went to see the doctor together. She had all the check-ups done. She is a healthy person. When everything was ready, we collected thirteen beautiful eggs from her. We had eleven embryos after the fertilization with my husband's sperms, and then we froze them. I had to get a physical check-up done again because I had been through so many operations. I was menopausal because of the medication. I had to be on another medication which would help me to have my period. After I had my period, they would check my hormone level. It had to be measured about three times before they found that I had the hormone. Then, we defrosted two embryos. The doctor suggested that the percentage of me getting pregnant was quite high so he did not want to defrost four embryos. If all of the four embryos worked, he would have to implant all four which he thought it was a waste.... Actually, he defrosted three but one dried out so we only had two left to put back. Initially, we thought that it would be twins. I was definitely pregnant but was not sure if it would be twins. A month later, we found that one of them dried out. The doctor felt relieved that it was not twins because he was worried about side effects that might occur. Everything went well. There were seven more eggs. Now, when the baby was in first year kinder, the doctor told me that I was ready to be pregnant again. This time, only three were defrosted because there is a big chance of me getting pregnant. We defrosted three ... failed one ... had two left ... then I was pregnant with another one so now, there are four left.

The doctor wants them to donate the excess eggs to other couples, however Ladda has not agreed: 'I just think that in case when they've grown up, they might come across each other and get married. It would be so horrible. The doctor comforted me that it was one out of a million chances that it would happen. Even so, I still don't want to be the one in those million chances so they still keep those eggs for me.'

Her younger sister has very little contact with her and her children 'She does not like kids so it's ok for me. She never comes and does not care.' She reflected that: 'The technology helps us to be more complete, otherwise it would only be just us the old couple. And we knew that the child we adopted has no love for us even though we love him so much.'

Ladda's story highlights many themes common to the participants in this study. Her complicated medical history is exacerbated by initial delays in seeking treatment, a poor system of referral, lack of initial knowledge about infertility treatment and encounters with unskilled doctors, iatrogenic treatment and poor communication. She pursues all opportunities to produce a biologically related child to feel 'more complete', finding adoption unsatisfactory and problematic. Across several years she endures a number of painful surgeries and interventions with different doctors, enmeshed in ever more complex technological interventions. Following repeated failure she finally pursues the assistance of an ova donor, in this case a relative, and through this finally gives birth successfully to two children.

As Frank van Balen and Marcia Inhorn point out (2002: 8), there is a paucity of cross-cultural material describing women's desires for motherhood. Further, because many previous studies of new reproductive technologies have tended to critique the patriarchal imperative for motherhood, they have sometimes failed to acknowledge the agency and strong desires and eagerness to birth and nurture children. Ladda's narrative highlights her agency and determination to overcome 'her destiny'. She underwent this treatment despite little support, she said even her husband was 'indifferent'. She makes clear reference to the assertion of her agency driven by her strong desire: 'I don't think anybody understood that I really wanted the baby. It was all me because I was the one who wanted the baby. I had to give myself the support because nobody thinks that it's good to have babies. They think that it's such a hassle.'

The boundaries of her treatment were dependent upon the technology available – once she found a clinic able to provide more technologically advanced interventions she pursued them. Throughout this narrative she describes her body in instrumental terms, as she described her 'dirty' tubes and the need to remove a tumour she compares her reproductive system as a set of failed parts. The interventions also lead her to view these failures in terms of the financial costs. Ultimately, the offer of money as compensation in exchange for her sister's assistance with an ova donation reflects this fragmented view of reproductive capacity and a growing commodification. But her pursuit of assisted reproduction has also left her with ongoing ethical issues, what to do with excess ova and the relationship with the ova donor.

Successful Pregnancy

For a fortunate minority, assisted reproduction results in a successful pregnancy. Couples expressed their disbelief and joy at positive pregnancy test results. But with pregnancy comes new anxieties. IVF pregnancies are treated as particularly special and vulnerable. In my sample of patients, four had experienced a successful pregnancy and birth through their treatment at the time of interview, one through the use of a surrogate. All couples interviewed described extra monitoring, care and testing during their pregnancies.

The return to the clinic visibly pregnant brings with it a sense of having moved on or graduated from couples that are continuing treatment. As Porn and Aruth noted: 'I felt envious when I was here and saw other patients who had succeeded. Now [that I am pregnant] I just want them to succeed and be happy like me. We understand and feel for them more because we had the problem before; for example, when our friends, who had the same problem, got pregnant, we were over the moon for them.'

The intense medicalization of conception and pregnancy with assisted reproduction is usually followed by a medicalized birth experience. Following successful pregnancies, most of the women I interviewed indicated they had been encouraged to give birth by elective caesarean section. The decision to undergo a caesarean is viewed by many obstetricians as ensuring a complication-free birth for the child in strictly controlled circumstances, a 'safer' alternative for such special IVF babies. Natural vaginal delivery is described as more 'risky'. Those carrying twins are rarely offered any alternative. An advantage of an elective caesarean is that it allows couples to choose the date and even time of the birth, an aspect important for those Thais with strong beliefs in astrology. The date and time of birth is believed to affect the child's future personality, fate and success in life. For example, Nit and Ton were going to consult an astrologer to choose the most auspicious day and time for the delivery of their twin boy and girl from a range of dates indicated as convenient by the doctor: 'We have an opportunity to pick the delivery date so we want to choose the best date for our baby.' Porn and Aruth were also pregnant with twins, and although they had hoped to have a natural childbirth – 'so I can recover quickly' – were recommended against doing so and were also going to have an elective caesarean. Ut and Khiat had booked a caesarean section because 'giving birth naturally is so tormenting', and also planned to bank the cord blood of their baby in case the child needed it in the future, as they felt it was unlikely the child would have any siblings.

Caesarean sections not only involve slower recovery for the mother, but also preclude women from undertaking traditional postpartum observances such as staying by the fire. As described above, apart from symbolically marking her new status as a mother, this practice, often glossed as 'mother roasting', is believed to dry out a new mother's womb, ensure the production of plentiful breast milk, enhance a woman's beauty and be prophylactic for her long-term reproductive health. Nuchnari was concerned that if she does have a caesarean, she would not have the opportunity to 'stay by the fire': 'The doctor told me that I would not be able to do that if I have a C-section. I want to though; I want to take herbal medicines. I want to follow the old traditions as it would be healthy for me. I want to have perfect and healthy milk. The doctor said that it would be ok if it was a natural birth [vaginal birth].'

Most women, however, were content to follow their doctor's recommendation, as in the case of Nut and Manit who also ended up with an elective caesarean section despite earlier expressing a wish to experience a 'natural' childbirth and to stay by the fire afterwards.

When to Stop

When asked, many patients interviewed claimed not to have considered when they might end treatment. They claimed they would persist 'as far as they could go' with the technology. Only a few had predetermined limits to their attempt with assisted technologies; they cited a range of limitations – money, the number of embryos stored, age limits – which would determine when they decided to cease treatment. Women such as Mon, for example, had decided to undergo treatment until she reached thirty-seven years of age; for Kwan, her limit was thirty-five. Pook's finances would limit her to undertake only two or three cycles. Porn and Aruth considered that they would continue treatment until they 'ran out of eggs'. Some patients such as Tuk said they would rely upon their doctor's advice. She explained: 'The doctor also said, "Go ahead. I will tell you when to stop. When there is no more chance, I'll let you know." And so my confidence increased. [He] gave me support.'

Many patients said they would try three times. Three is a particularly auspicious magic number in Buddhist Thailand, coinciding with the Three Jewels of Buddhism: the Buddha, the Dharma and the Sangha; and the Three Pillars of Thailand: the Monarchy, Religion and the Nation. When asked how many times they would try IUI, Daeng, for instance, replied: 'It might be my personal preference from being a Buddhist. I would actually try once and accept that it's my destiny, but I don't mind trying three times. It's still okay at my age to try but I would not do any more than three times.'

However, some patients seem either not to have been told they had reached the limits of the technology or had refused to heed such advice. The 'never-enough' quality of assisted reproductive technologies has been commented upon by Margarete Sandelowski (1991). Ying gave a stunning example of this when asked when she would contemplate finishing treatment. At forty-five years old and with no financial constraints, she had already undergone eight years of various treatments and IVF cycles. Only one doctor had had the temerity to suggest she should cease treatment, advice she rejected by moving to another clinic. She was now using an egg donor/surrogate. She now suggests that the age of her surrogate may determine when she stops: 'In another two years the surrogate will be twenty-six or twenty-seven years old and then I will say enough and then if we don't have a child then that's enough. That will demonstrate truly that we won't have a child – it isn't our fate to have a child. But having said that I'm not sure, there might be cloning by then and I might try that.'

Conclusions

The clinical space is liminal (van Gennep 1960: 1), a space of denial, discipline and technological rituals. Within the clinic and through its practices and interactions with staff, infertile couples are defined as patients and they take on ambiguous new identities as parents-to-be. Embryos are regarded and spoken of as future children. Although presented in scientific terms, I suggest that the practices and technical interventions cast their own enchantment. During treatment patients devote themselves to disciplined routines and protocols, undergo bodily interventions and transformations, submit themselves to strict sexual discipline and in many cases do so within conditions of secrecy. As in other liminal spaces time is reorganized within the clinic, with bodily rhythms regulated through pharmaceuticals and hormones and measured and choreographed in terms of reproductive age, cycles and doctors' appointments. Yet there are no guarantees that careful observance of the rituals will produce a successful transition to parenthood. For all the presentation of assisted reproduction as science, manipulated and mediated by expert clinicians, mystery and miracles remain.

In this chapter I have described the processes of medicalization, visualization and monitoring and figurative dissection and discipline of the body central to the practice of assisted reproduction. Deborah Wilson Lowry (2004) suggests we might describe such practices as a form of 'surveillant assemblage', surveillance centred on securing knowledge and making visible human bodies through technological processes. As seen across this chapter, assisted reproduction involves the monitoring and distribution of information about infertile women and men. The focus upon an abstraction of the body and embryonic body, the significance and fetishization of sophisticated machinery and its application across middle class and elite women and men operate within these settings. The dissection of the infertile body through testing and visualization results in the formation of a 'data double' of the patient and of embryonic material even before birth – a 'flesh-technology-information amalgam' or cyborg (Haggerty and Ericson 2000: 611; also Haraway 1991). The abstraction and creation of a data double allows for interventions and monitoring at various levels, by additional tests, the development of further technologies, perceived imperfection of the foetus, reduction to statistical level allowing the monitoring of clinics themselves.

Yet we should not read these practices as only involving the domination of patients. The Thai women and men of this study speak in similar terms to those observed by Franklin: 'IVF pronatalism is narrated as an aggressive pursuit of an elusive goal in which women are warriors, with battle scars attesting to their bravery on an epic quest for a child of their own. Passivity is not a virtue in the world of achieved conception' (1997: 162). It is clear from the interviews presented here that many women and men participate in and collaborate with these processes; living with the tensions and contradictions such objectification, visualisation and monitoring involves. Evident in these couples descriptions is that the experience of IVF, its success and failures, involve not only notions of discipline, with blame, anxiety and guilt as responses to failure, but also a complex mix of feelings of hope, self-satisfaction, nobility and achievement. Added to these are parables of other couples that struggled through numerous cycles over many years, eventually to achieve a successful live birth. If despite the sacrifices undergone, no child results, then couples speak of accepting their fate or destiny as childless. In this way the process is imbued with a noble sense of a cause. Rayna Rapp once described couples using new assisted reproductive technologies as 'moral pioneers' (Rapp 1987). Like pioneers their journey is predicated on a utopian vision of the future, and like many pioneers the realities often fall short of their hopes.

Chapter 5

The Clinical Ensemble

> Music and melodies are composed by the note and scale. It requires much imagination and is very difficult to compose. However, music is behind the success of the songs sung. And the songs are behind the success of a singer. Perfect music will make the song beautiful. A beautiful song will make the singer sing well, with emotion and become successful and famous. The singer is someone who simply recites the lyric and sings along to the melodies that someone else has composed. They use only a little bit of their abilities but become successful and famous among the general public. The composers contribute more but become less successful, less famous, and less well known. – Teerapong, *Khon Mii Luuk Yaak Khon Yak Mii Luuk* (Those Who Have Difficulties Having a Baby / Those Who Want to Have a Baby), 250–51

In this chapter I introduce some of the health providers involved in assisted reproduction and explore what is defined as good quality of care by patients. In all the private and public clinics that I visited or conducted observations, health staff were very busy, working long hours with large caseloads. The staff of infertility clinics describe their work in special terms as a vocation, not just technical expertise. They tend to speak very positively of the technologies and encourage persistence among their patients in the hope of eventual success. They recognize the significance of their work as arbiters of the stuff of life itself.

Within infertility clinics, the act of conception becomes a mediated enterprise requiring medical expertise (Bonaccorso 2009). The clinic itself is a physical space where conception becomes explicit and nonintimate and, as suggested in the previous chapter, it is also a liminal space in which parents-to-be undergo rituals as they forge a new status.

One doctor described assisted reproduction as a 'tripartite affair', between a woman, man and doctor, but in fact there are a cast of other actors involved, including nurses, auxiliaries, embryologists and other lab staff. In the quote above from the book *Khon mii luuk yaak khon yaak mii luuk* (คนมีลูกยาก คนอยากมีลูก; Those who have difficulties having a baby / Those who want to have a baby) the relationship between patients and medical staff is likened to the production of music by a singer and musicians following musical notation, who must all practice and work together harmoniously to produce a fine sound. While some parts of the collaboration become famous, the others also contribute greatly to the success. The doctor in this same book is described as a 'friend who means well' (Teerapong 2001). Similarly, Thompson (2005) writes of the 'ontological choreography' required to make parents and a viable embryo. Numerous actors, including nurses, doctors, patients and others, must choreograph precisely timed biological acts (injection of hormones, the production of gametes, the timing of transfer) within the clinic. As Thompson notes, this also increasingly involves the 'strategic naturalization' of third parties, so-called reproductive assistors, gestational surrogates and gamete donors and resultant new forms of kinship.

In the second part of this chapter I examine what patients think and expect of their doctors. They have very specific ideas about what constitutes a good IVF doctor. Although to a certain degree patients' impressions of their doctors is partly determined by the success of their treatment, it is also clear that patients value good interpersonal skills, communication and personalized care from their doctors. Many patients have stories of paternalistic, demeaning and arrogant treatment at the hands of certain doctors, and in some cases technical incompetence and even fraud. In some cases these are IVF doctors, in others, nonspecializing gynaecologists who intervene surgically or fail to recognize the necessity for referral to an assisted reproductive clinic, causing delays and in some cases further damaging their patients' fertility. Such experiences can cause patients to forego or cease treatment, constituting yet another constraint upon their access to these technologies. In other cases, patients moved between several clinics and doctors in their quests for care. This is of interest given that, for the most part, doctor-patient relationships in Thailand involve a power dynamic in which the doctor is viewed as authoritative and his (usually male) opinion unquestioned. I examine what patients say about their doctors and what motivates them to swap doctors.

Running throughout these accounts is the tension that exists between public and private practice. Such is the demand for services that, apart from the major public hospitals, assisted reproductive treatments are now available in most large private hospitals. In addition a number of doctors or consortiums of doctors have started their own stand-alone specialist infertility clinics. According to the Thai ART registry, at the time of my research there were thirty clinics licensed to provide assisted reproductive treatments in Thailand, evidence of the rapid global penetration of new reproductive technologies into Thailand since 1989. Three-quarters of these clinics are clustered in Bangkok while other centres are located in the major regional towns. Yet, as described in the introduction, these clinics do not come close to covering the demand for services (Vutyavanich et al. 2011). Tensions exist between what is described by doctors in altruistic terms as their 'public service' and the profits available in private practice. Many doctors involved in assisted reproduction in fact straddle both, and increasing privatization of assisted reproduction within public hospitals is also blurring the distinction.

Careers in Vivo

I was walking in the market on my way to the clinic when I received a phone call informing me that once again Dr X would have to cancel our appointment for an interview because of a patient issue that had arisen. I had tried several times to arrange an interview with Dr X, the head of one of the public infertility clinics in which I was doing my research. Dr X had generously allowed me to sit in his clinic for several months, interviewing patients in a private meeting room. He had been an enthusiastic supporter of the research and had assisted me in introductions to other infertility specialists, many of whom were former students of his. I was introduced to him months before and we had some short informal chats, but I wanted to have some dedicated time for a taped interview to ask him about some of the things I had observed and heard in my interviews with patients. I knew how overworked and overscheduled he was, so I fully understood his need to cancel our appointment. But it was to be one of the frustrations of my research in infertility clinics that opportunities to formally interview the doctors themselves were to prove rare. I learned to ask as much as possible and be polite in my initial meetings in clinics as I knew that I might not have a second chance. I never doubted the main reason was because of the time pressures these doctors face. Although most acute in public practice, both private and public specialists carry enormous caseloads. Most public specialists also maintain after-hours private practices and many also have teaching and administrative responsibilities.

Because the IVF community of doctors is so small, to protect anonymity here I provide an overview drawn from the doctors I worked with rather than give individual case studies. All the doctors I met with were experienced in the field, usually with over ten years' and in some cases over twenty years' experience with IVF. Most had spent periods of study overseas to develop their skills in assisted reproduction in the United States, England and Australia and maintained professional associations with clinics and specialists in those countries. Indeed, some clinics actively promoted their ties with overseas clinics as prestigious evidence of the quality and international standard of their service. On the whole, the doctors I met were dedicated and passionate about their work, they enjoyed the intellectual challenges it posed and the scientific interest, but they also saw their work as involving a special relationship with a patient, in which they facilitated a new life and new family. One of the doctors I worked with had himself had used the technology to form his family. In his case he said he felt he had special empathy with his patients and understood their needs.

The Thai book '*Yak pen mae khae khad jai*': Mommy's story' (Threechana and Pimonsing 2004) contains a number of comments from doctors on their work in assisted reproduction. In this book, another doctor, Dr ML Thongthithongyai, also comments that he used assisted reproduction:

> I am also the one who has problem with infertility and my babies are test tube babies. They are my best gift ever. Now I'm fifty. In the next ten years, I might be dead or can't work anymore. However, while I live and while I can work, I will do my best for my family, friends, and society. My children are my inspiration/encouragement for me to do these good things. I'm proud to be able to fulfil my patients' dreams, to make them happy, and to help them have their perfect families.

All the doctors I met were extremely busy with multiple demands upon their time. One doctor described his working hours:

> I come in before seven AM every morning. I am the first to sign in and the last person to sign out. I am the one who always opens the door.

> ... I have to come in everyday and make sure if everything is working well because even a small thing can cause other problems. I even check the floor. It creates a culture as well; all other staff and nurses start at seven AM to help me. I come in first to check that everything is ready.... Secondly, I never take a day off; I work even on weekends. I think this is the core; determination and dedication to my work.... No matter whether one practices medicine or does any kind of work, you have to be able to answer certain questions so that you can succeed; first of all, do you have seven days available for work in a week? If you say 'no' and treat it as a hobby, I think you better give up. You have to ask yourself if you have 365 [days] per year to do the job.

Doctors were not always satisfied with the limitations of their role, the heavy caseloads and limited time they had with each patient, nor the difficulties and frustrations of using technologies which carried no guarantees of success. Despite their best efforts, at times some couples defied all attempts and doctors admitted that sometimes they simply did not know why cycles failed. The hardest thing was to watch couples repeatedly fail and not be able to assist them. As one doctor commented:

> As human beings we always try to be most complete and successful even though we have developed it [the assisted technology] to be successful from zero per cent to 25–30 per cent.... It might not be conclusive as yet but there are still many issues that we want to eliminate such as abnormalities in chromosomes that cause miscarriage. ... I don't see any [scientific] breakthroughs in the near future. The only thing I can see is trying to eliminate problems that will occur to embryos.

Although he suggested most doctors are fascinated with the technical challenges of fertility treatment, he noted that it was important for doctors to also recognize and take care of their patients' mental health: 'It's not just the physical side we have to care for, mental care is also important. It's like we produce a tailor-made shirt, not just selling in bulk.'

As noted in chapter 1, the status of assisted reproduction has rapidly changed. Experienced doctors commented upon the early neglect of their specialty: the difficulties in convincing hospital authorities of the need for assisted reproduction services and the poor resourcing they experienced. One doctor suggested that originally his programme did not attract a lot of support. Infertility treatment was not seen as a high priority and as elective rather than necessary health care, and they experienced funding difficulties at first as the hospital management 'didn't see the importance of it'. Over time this had changed, and the recent proliferation of private clinics was in part due to the recognition by hospitals of the demand and profitability of these services, as one doctor noted, an IVF patient comes repeatedly over a long period of time for treatment; they are healthy but frequent clients, profitable for hospitals. All patients had to pay out of pocket for their treatment.

In some cases doctors had abandoned the Thai public health system, working exclusively for the private sector or within their own private facilities. Some doctors are quite entrepreneurial and their clinics are advertised widely and become well known through their use by high-profile personalities. This tension between working in public and private settings was commented upon by some public clinic doctors who criticized some other practitioners for being overly concerned about making money rather than caring for their patients, citing unethical practice, inflated claims of success and over-servicing as issues within the profession. The relative lack of regulation was seen as contributing to these problems, a problem soon to be addressed by legislation.

The doctors in private hospital clinics described their choice not to work within the public sector as about being able to provide good quality of care for their patients. They felt that overcrowding and

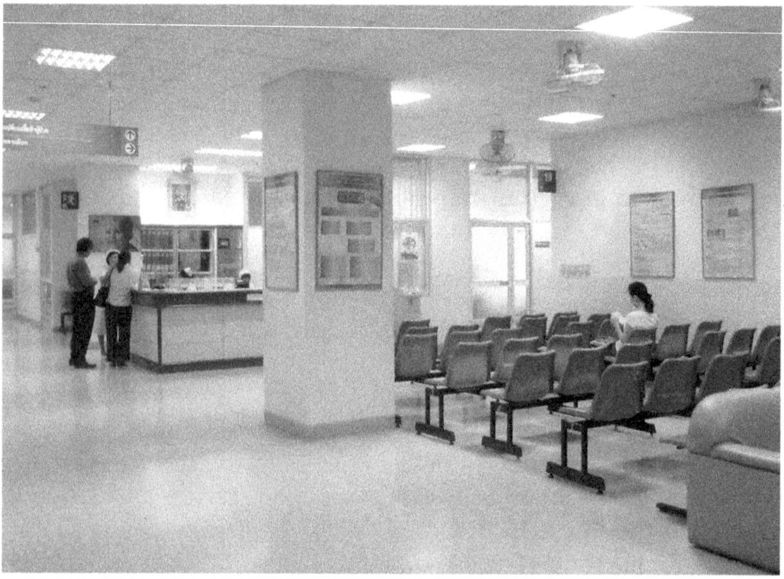

FIGURE 5.1. The waiting area of an infertility clinic in one of the public hospitals.

rushed consultations of public clinics interfere with high-quality care. They also suggested that private hospitals tended to have the resources to invest in better-equipped laboratories and that the higher compensation ensured they worked with excellent nursing and laboratory staff.

Yet such differentiations between the public and private sector are becoming increasingly irrelevant within Thailand as more public hospitals, including even Siriraj Hospital, the oldest medical school in the country, develop medical complexes to service private patients and compete with the private sector. Staff from the public hospital rotate to the private wing for a number of hours each week. These initiatives are seen to address the trend for doctors to leave the overcrowded public sector for better compensation and form part of the increasing privatization of Thailand's health services more generally. Given that many of the costs involved in assisted reproductive treatment such as the prices of hormones are similar, the difference in costs of treatment equates to differences in service. As will be shown in the discussion below, private patients expect and receive more time with their doctors, more personalized treatment and higher staffing levels. Public patients in general have shorter consultations, may see junior physicians and ancillary staff for their appointments, and are faced with queues and long waits due to the heavy caseloads of their doctors. But as will see, there is a flow of Thai patients between public and private clinics. This is because public university teaching hospitals are highly prestigious institutions whose staff are highly regarded and have usually been at the forefront of the technology in Thailand. Their large caseloads also mean that doctors there are very experienced and usually have good success rates. Likewise, most public specialists also have private clinics after hours, and in some cases patients will transfer between the two, blurring the distinctions between public and private practice.

The Embryologist

Although much attention is focussed upon IVF doctors, in reality the success of any assisted reproduction treatment depends heavily on the experience, skill and quality of the laboratory services. Within the laboratory, the embryologist is a specialist laboratory scientist responsible for the care, growth and selection of embryos before they are transferred back into a human body. I interviewed two of the embryologists in one public and one private clinic. Both were dedicated to their jobs and spoke of the challenges it posed and felt a sense of vocation and responsibility in their roles.

Within the public clinic it was difficult to get to interview Achan Noi, as she is always tremendously busy and would flash a smile as she walked rapidly through a room between the laboratory and consulting rooms. Achan Noi formerly worked in the genetics laboratory of this hospital and was asked to head up the embryology and andrology laboratory when IVF started at the hospital in 1987. Her career has spanned thirty years and although she could find better-paid jobs in the private sector, she prefers working at a prestigious public teaching hospital. She said the clinic has difficulties attracting embryologists due to the better pay in the private sector. Likewise, they have a lot of difficulty getting nursing staff for the clinic as the wages are considerably higher and the working conditions not so crowded at private hospitals; she said nurses and staff that do come here must be quite devoted and committed to this hospital and public work.

Although she has been working in IVF for many years, Achan Noi still gets 'very happy' when she sees an embryo undergoing cell division and gets disappointed to learn that a 'grade A, beautiful' egg has not resulted in a pregnancy: 'I have to remind myself that it is not just about the egg but other factors such as the lining of the womb etc. I know the patients start to stress [when they are not successful] but I feel I have done the very best in terms of the lab science.' Achan Noi gave me a tour of the laboratory and proudly showed off the latest purchase, a new micromanipulator microscope for the delicate ICSI procedures. She showed me the corridors of the clinic lined with large storage containers (see figure 5.2).

> Our clinic has not yet destroyed any embryos from fifteen years of operation. We are storing them and trying to contact patients to see if they want to retain them but if they can't contact them then they are currently retaining them as they have owners, they have life [*mi jaokhong, mi chiwit*]. However, after fifteen years we are running out of storage space and so something will have to be done. I think the lab will begin stem cell research, currently we are setting things up but again it [stem cell research] will be with the permission of the patients.

We passed through to the surgery where IUI and laparoscopic procedures take place, ova are collected and embryos transferred. Three surgical beds stand parallel to each other, curtains dividing them from each other. We spoke further about her excitement when she sees eggs divide, the expense of imported high-quality growth media and the future plans to move and expand the clinic.

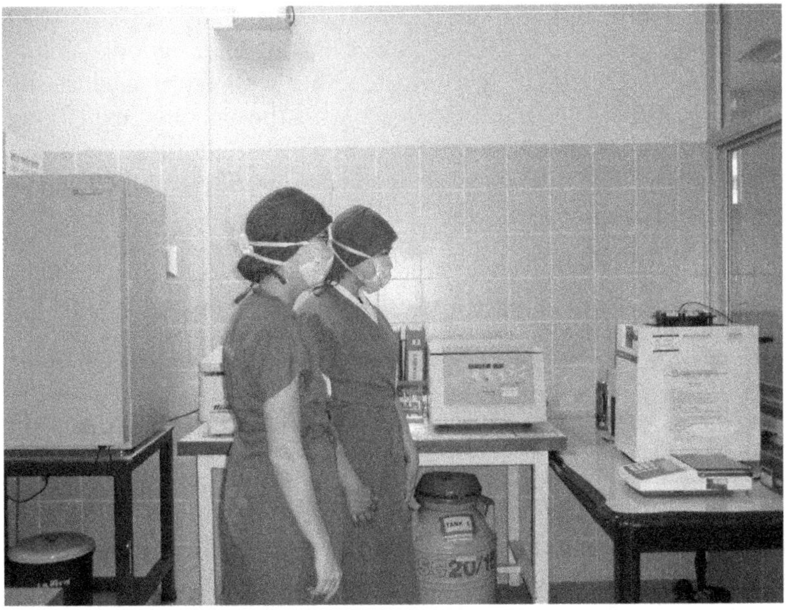

FIGURE 5.2. The author and embryologist having a tour of the laboratory in a public hospital.

Khun Nop worked in a private hospital. She trained as a lab scientist and started working in assisted reproduction in 1993 in a private clinic that now conducts about eighty ovarian stimulation cycles per year:

> They could see how I worked and my attention to detail in addition to my love of working in a lab. I needed to practice until I became skilful enough so that I could actually do the job. I started from working with sperms. I had to work on controlling small instruments such as little glass pokers and rubber stoppers. Everything is so small so I have to work via using a microscope. After I had a good experience with preparing sperms, then, I could move on to dealing with eggs. I had to learn how each piece of equipment worked and how to maintain and look after the equipment. There are differences between being a spectator and being an operator. Everything looked so easy when I was a spectator but when I really do the work myself, I have to think about the next steps all the time. It is a hand-made job and we have to work against time in which the skill comes with experience.

Like Achan Noi, Khun Nop also described her work as a vocation: 'I am pleased that I can help people who have infertility problems. If you come in contact with them, you will know how much they are suffering. I will think of them every single step of my work. I cannot *just* do my work. I treat this as if I was looking after my own child.'

As the embryologist in a private clinic with fewer clients, she spends considerable time in contact with the patients, explaining the steps in the lab and phoning them daily to inform them about the progress of the embryos prior to transfer. She emphasized the importance of communication and service:

> I think it should be the warmth that patients can feel. Services provided by doctors and nurses in Thailand are quite impressive. Partly, I think doctors in Thailand spend more time with their patients more and by nature; Thais tend to smile and be more sympathetic to others. It is important for patients in this field to have plenty of moral support. Sometimes, a doctor does not need to be brilliant but patients are happy that their doctors look after them very well.

I was surprised that unlike other labs I visited, this lab is kept dark lit by red light like a photography darkroom and close to body temperature; she explained that this was to create conditions as close to that inside the human body as possible for the gametes and embryos when they are being manipulated within the lab. I wondered how staff could bear to work for long periods in the heat. She explained that staff take regular breaks as they need to be able to concentrate. She proudly showed me the dishes in the incubator growing embryos and the micromanipulators. I watched in fascination as one of the staff members practiced by injecting a sperm into a damaged ova; at another machine a staff member was undertaking a sperm count, counting each spermatozoa within a grid overlaid on a fresh sample. She explained the lab's procedures for ensuring there were no mix-ups of gametes in the lab: they only worked on one couple's samples at a time and they carefully rechecked the labels. After we left the lab she described her delight and intellectual curiosity in her work, which she described as both work and a form of making merit (*tham bun*).

The Counsellor

Only one clinic in which I studied provided dedicated nurse-counsellors. Nurse Toy is one of three counsellors available in person and by phone at a private clinic. After graduating as a nurse she has worked at a number of hospitals and institutes for over thirteen years. 'Initially, I was not that interested in IVF. There was a vacancy in the department which I successfully applied for, and once

I started working I found that I enjoyed it and I have been working in it ever since.' She works closely with the doctors at the clinic and has learned her counselling skills largely through them, although she also attends training courses so that she can understand the various procedures. She would like to undertake some training overseas but needs to improve her English before she can do so. Nurse Toy is thirty-nine years old. She stated: 'I would use it [the technology] with myself. At the moment, I am not married yet but once I get married, with my age, I think I will need the technology to help me.' We asked Nurse Toy what patients come to ask her about:

> Mostly, [patients] would expect to know straight away what their chances of success are. First issues, they want to know if their case is a difficult or rare case, and whether there will be any complications. While having their procedures, they want to make sure if they are doing the right things or what they supposed to do. There are a lot of questions until the end of the procedure. Most of their worries involve their expectations ... high expectations. Even though we have told the patients that it is not one hundred per cent guaranteed, they still expect that this [IVF] can be the way that leads them to success.

Nurse Toy sees the patients before they see a doctor:

> I start from when they come in. I advise them about preparing themselves before an appointment with a doctor. I will explain to them what to expect in the process, step by step, such as what kinds of tests need to be done first. Once we have the results, the doctor would decide the method of treatment. Then, I have to explain and confirm the steps of the treatment again, to ensure that the patient fully understands the process even though the doctor has explained to them already. I would see if they still have any more questions regarding the treatment. Sometimes, the patients can't think of the questions to ask while they are with the doctor, so the nurse has to explain step by step again.... Once we discuss about certain things already, it does not mean that we would not come back to those again. We still follow up with the patient every step until the case is finished.... Working in my area, I would love to have a closer relationship with our patients. There are only three counsellors dealing with all patients, so it's difficult for us to get to know them at a deeper level. I would like the patients to feel more comfortable talking to us and feel that they have someone to go to. With the number of patients, we can only provide them information about the treatment's process.

Nurse Toy or one of the other counsellors is on hand for patients to talk with anytime during their treatment. The hardest part of her job is counselling people after repeated failures. She also feels bad when patients elect to undergo selective reductions of multiple embryos: 'I don't feel good about it but each has their own reasons for their decision. We have to accept that it's their lives and they have the right to do what they wish for.' Unlike the public clinic described above, this private clinic will dispose of excess embryos if no longer required, although she says it is a hard decision and sometimes patients come for advice. Each year the clinic sends out a letter asking if the patients wish to continue storing their excess embryos or whether to dispose of them: 'The patient needs to sign a consent form to authorize that we can destroy the embryos, and then it would be the lab's responsibility to follow the patient's instructions. ... I personally do feel that they are live cells but it's a patient's individual right so it's up to them.'

The Nurse

Nurse Sriubol has been working as a nurse at the public hospital for twenty-five years and in the public clinic since 2001. Apart from her nursing role assisting doctors in procedures, her role within the clinic is largely administrative. Because she is on the front desk she also provides advice, information and counselling to patients, who tend to turn to her due to her experience and seniority for explanations of procedures and medications: 'I like working in this field because I get to see patients with all emotions; happy and sad. I get to be there for them. Some patients are really determined to work with the doctor. They came to us with their infertility problems and we try to investigate the cause of the problem with doctors. Causes might not be found for some patients, they get frustrated and do not come back. I feel that we still could not reach to them and I just want to know what to do to help them succeed.'

We asked what stood out as the best and worst experiences of working in assisted reproduction and she said that she was touched by one case where a woman succeeded in falling pregnant after three years of continuous attempts. In contrast, she found a case when one woman gave up IVF once she reached menopause very disappointing. She said she tends to counsel women to continue treatment if at all possible. Nurse Sriubol has herself had treatment for infertility at this same clinic using the GIFT technique. Ten years ago she gave birth to a daughter: 'Because the aim of having a married life is to have an heir ... I used this treatment here myself.... It was not so difficult; one cycle per month. I just kept trying and had a limit that if I reached a certain age and it decreased the chance of success, I would come to terms with it and stop trying.'

She continued treatment for two years before succeeding. She now draws upon her experience when counselling patients; she doesn't tell every patient she has had treatment, 'only with patients I am more familiar with or patients who have already tried many times'. She says her advice to patients is 'to follow through the process progressively. It does not matter where you decided to have this kind of treatment, not necessary to be here (at this clinic), patients just need to follow through.'

Relationship between Medical Staff and Patients

As noted earlier, doctors hold positions of high status and respect in Thailand, their opinions are rarely questioned and they tend to be viewed as beneficent patrons to submissive clients rather than service providers to health consumers. Patients generally defer to a doctor and would rarely challenge him or her, which would cause a loss of face for both parties (Klausner 1993). Bonaccorso (2009: 72) notes in the Italian clinics in which she worked that clinicians are viewed as holding 'exceptional expertise with which they control the procreative project and possibly make it happen' and exercise 'great authority' with patients because of their knowledge. For example, Naa commented of her doctor: 'Here I am satisfied with the treatment. I believe everything the doctor says. Whatever he says I believe. I feel he is the only one who can help me. Whatever he recommends is beneficial. Although he doesn't speak a lot. You have to ask him. Because sometimes we wonder about things that we shouldn't wonder about and the doctor doesn't tell us.' Predictably, couples who were successful in becoming pregnant expressed enormous admiration for their doctor: 'We are very thankful to the doctor. He is like another father to the baby. If it was not because of the doctor, we would not be here as a parents today' (Ut and Khiat).

Strict hierarchies were evident in all the clinics in which I worked. IVF specialists had the highest status, followed by their medical staff and head of the laboratory. Nurses deferred to doctors and had their own hierarchy based on seniority. Various auxiliary staff members occupied the lowest-status roles within the clinics. Depending on their position status and wealth, patients generally defer to both doctors and senior nurses.

As will be discussed below, patients largely chose their doctors on the basis of their reputations, with expectations of a straightforward course of treatment and eventual success. They often relied on the referrals from friends, relatives and work colleagues who have experienced successful treatment as evidence of the skill of the doctor. Just as Bonaccorso (2009: 72–73) describes for Italian clinics, Thai patients place trust and faith in their doctors and display high levels of dependency upon them, meticulously following their advice. The general lack of familiarity with intensive medical care and technicalities of reproductive treatment combined with the strong desires of both patients and practitioners for the technologies to work makes for complex relationships between doctors and patients. As can be seen in the nurses' comments above, patients are urged to not give up hope and to continue to have faith in their doctors and the technologies and to continue to fight (*su*) and persist.

As described in chapter 3 patients come to realize over time that assisted reproductive treatments are not straightforward and the chances of success are low, leading to a gradual disillusionment with the limitations of reproductive medicine (Becker 2000: 123) and a tendency to 'shop around' for other clinics or other doctors. Medical staff generally agree that all IVF services in Thailand were 'pretty much the same as each other', as one nurse put it, in terms of their standards of care and success rates, although they differed in the services they could offer, most notably the availability of ICSI and PGD services. Yet patients affirm their belief in the superiority of some doctors and clinics over others.

Patients' Views of Quality of Care

Good quality of care was defined by patients not in terms of pregnancy success rates, but in terms of: communication, empathy and personalized care from their doctor, sufficient time for consultations and the opportunity to ask questions, respectful treatment from nursing staff, a lack of excessive waiting times or overcrowding, the opportunity to have concerns answered by phone by a doctor or nursing staff after hours and communication from the embryologist.

Having a doctor who was a good communicator was highly valued by patients. Ut (age thirty-one) and her husband Khiat (thirty-two) underwent three ICSI/IVF cycles at a private clinic and were now pregnant with their first child. I asked them what they thought of their doctor:

> We think of the doctor as if he was an angel. [We are impressed] even with the way he speaks. I had an experience with a doctor in the area we live, he was not very nice. This doctor is so positive. He encourages us every step of the way. He does not make it to be a serious issue for us at all. We can call the doctor from our home no matter how insignificant the problem is. We get to speak to the doctor almost every time. He even gave us his private phone number and would call us back when he's busy. When we failed again the second time, the doctor was also stressed. The doctor was worried for us because he thought that our case should have been an easy case. He helped us until we have succeeded. He was so wonderful with us. No matter what kind of questions we have, he would have answers for us. Besides, whenever we called him with any concerns, he would make us feel relaxed and calm.

Only private patients reported that they were offered after-hours numbers to call a nurse or doctor for advice if they had difficulties with their injections or hormone regimes. In addition, in private clinics couples received regular updates during the cell division growth stages in vitro. Mot had changed doctors because of her previous doctor's poor communication skills:

> One of the reasons we chose this doctor is because he is really calm. He would answer questions or explain things in details. I had an experience with a doctor at P Private Hospital. The doctor there did not explain much. He might think that it was too complicated to explain and we might not understand. We feel good with the doctor here, we can call to ask questions any time.

The ability to ask questions was linked to the length of time in consultations. Many patients in public hospitals complained about the limited consultation time with their doctor. This inhibited them from asking too many questions of their doctor. The power differential between a doctor and patient further discourages much active questioning from patients. As a result, many expressed confusion about their treatment or test results. For example, Nut and Manit were waiting for the results of a prenatal serum genetic test but were confused about what the results might mean: 'Dr did explain but he didn't say much. We must ask him. The main problem is doctors hardly talk. Not only this department but every department [in the hospital].' Likewise, a public patient, Phen, explained that she had little idea about her treatment or the steps involved. She said she was satisfied with her treatment but would like more information from her doctor or nurses about what to expect:

> My suggestion would be that if patients come to consult about something they should let them know in advance that this is what the doctor is going to do. That with this technique the doctor will do this ... this is what will happen next.... It is like patients come and just sit wondering and then enter the room. And then there is the [intravaginal] ultrasound. How would I know what the ultrasound would be like? I came here the first time. And you are left to imagine it yourself, so this is the ultrasound! I would like the doctor to advise that these are the steps because I came and then was puzzled and then get changed and then 'What's next?' I tried to find a nurse to ask what was going to happen next and she said 'Go and sit, go and sit right here!' And what will they do to me next? I would like them to advise me to let me know in advance about what I have to do next.

Because of the limited time with her doctor, Faa tended to ask the nurses at the public clinic for information: 'They [nurses] can explain things although they talk a little fast. If we don't understand we have to repeat our questions as they use medical terms. ... I know that they have limited time, so we only ask what is really necessary.'

Lek was openly critical of the public clinic where she was being treated. In particular she was annoyed that she might only see a junior intern or auxiliary staff at her appointment rather than the specialist. She had moved to this clinic on the basis of the specialist's reputation and felt that the doctor should see her: 'I would like it to be that if we get the treatment with this doctor then it should be them [the same doctor] all the time. I don't want to see different doctors.' Despite travelling far to attend her appointments, she would end up with very little time with the doctor, and often didn't feel she had sufficient time to ask questions: 'Very little time, less than five minutes. It's like the doctor has cases outside [private cases] and OPD [outpatient department]. I understand but the doctor should also understand that we have come from so far, we have travelled. I would like to ask things that I would like to know.'

Public hospital treatment involved enduring long waiting times, overcrowding and limited appointments. I observed in one public clinic that during busy morning clinics there would be too few seats for the patients – often people would be forced to stand to wait for their appointment or procedure. Tum and Bunmi commented that although the infertility clinic was less crowded than other parts of the hospital, 'they say that here if you exhale it will be inhaled by someone else. There are so many patients; there is no way the air can go through!' Mon described the public clinic she attends:

The place has too few seats and a lot of patients. On the one side is the maternity clinic and on this side the infertility clinic, for those who are sensitive they would feel a bit uncomfortable with that [seeing heavily pregnant women going to the maternal foetal medicine clinic opposite]. The seats here are not comfortable. The other side [in maternity] looks more comfortable and there are more seats. The number of service providers is less than the customers. I feel the number of patients is increasing. Some weeks there are not enough seats and some people have to stand because they come as a couple.

As large institutions, the public hospitals had complex appointment, referral and payment systems that confused patients. Even finding the right building and clinic could be difficult. Ladda (age forty-five, pregnant with IVF/donor egg) noted that at the public clinic she attended, people had to queue to get in for their clinic appointments. They needed to arrive early and receive tickets and must wait for their number to be called before they can attend an appointment. She had been warned beforehand about how the system worked. For people who were not familiar with this particular hospital's systems, it could mean long delays and lost opportunities to see a doctor: 'If I did not know anyone there, I would have to be in a queue, waiting since five AM to get a docket [to get in]. Staff at the department downstairs have very poor manners. Let's say … if I got there and the quota for the day had been filled, I would have to wait another week.' She found the system confusing and the administrative and nursing staff rude:

Staff in a public hospital are not very good. I was called 'crazy' by staff downstairs! Doctors and assistants [in the clinic] are good but staff downstairs are so old and mean. They judged that I was crazy because I did not know the [hospital's] procedures. For me, I am more used to a shopping mall because I always go shopping. It's not like I go to a hospital all the time. If we are not sick we will not go to a hospital.

She recounted the difficulties she had encountered when she was required to undergo tests and surgery as part of her treatment:

The staff asked me when the bed was for and I told them that I did not know. Before I could tell them that I had a plan to move to Bangkok-Christian Hospital for the surgery, they gave me attitudes and said that I was crazy. They did not understand how the person on their right mind would not know when she would have her operation. Blah, blah, blah. I had to pretend that it was my fault and apologize to them because I was afraid that I would not be able to get the heart checked-up on time. They assumed that I was crazy and even walked

> away, pretending to do other things. I was so scared because I really wanted to have a baby. I knew that they weren't doctors but I called them doctors just to make them feel good. I kept apologizing to them so they could get things done for me. They snappishly did it as if they were doing me a big favour. I was so upset about it. Moreover, I had to get my lung x-rayed at another department. I dealt with this young staff member who wore a black and white uniform, looked like a student. The young staff member told me to go into a room and wait for another staff member to do the x-ray. I asked her if I needed to do anything else and she told me bluntly just to get into the room. I just wanted to know if I needed to take off my top. I did not tell this to the doctors because I knew that they were so busy already. I did not want to annoy them with these little issues. Once finished, the staff just walked off without saying anything. I did not know if that was all I needed to do or where else I needed to go. I was told to wait so I was waiting in a white gown for about an hour and nobody came to tell me anything. I could not remember who she was because there were so many people in black and white uniform. I asked another staff around there but she had no idea. She asked me which staff I dealt with and I could not tell. This is Hospital C. It's just so, so bad.

Disenchantment: Changing Doctors

Frustrations with poor communication, overcrowding and repeated failed cycles lead many patients to change doctors and clinics in the hope of success elsewhere. Although doctors suggested that there was little difference in the standards of care across the various clinics in Thailand, patients suggested there could be a marked difference in protocols and skill between doctors and expressed the belief that finding the 'right' fit was important for successful treatment. Ying, for example, had undergone treatment across many years at six different private and public clinics in Bangkok without success. Her case is discussed in greater detail in chapter 9. Despite being counselled by one doctor to forego further treatment, she continued to seek treatment. She considered herself an expert in the various drug regimens favoured by different doctors and had become a savvy and critical consumer. Although hers was an extreme example, she was by no means exceptional. Many of the patients I interviewed had switched doctors at some stage. Most had histories of multiple failed attempts. Poy was typical in that she had tried 'IUI, GIFT, ICSI two times and last time last year and then moved' to another clinic. 'Our attempt at ICSI resolved that we won't have a baby, so we thought we wouldn't, but then changed our mind. Let's change and try a new doctor [instead].' Within a country where the power differential is marked between doctors and patients and doctors' opinions are rarely questioned or criticized, such movement between doctors speaks of the disenchantment many patients experience towards the medical profession and the technology when treatment fails.

Over-servicing and iatrogenic treatment were also experienced by some patients. Apart from the pain and trauma of unnecessary or ineffective surgeries, such experiences made them mistrust the medical profession. As described in chapter 1, occasionally the media describe cases of fraud and malpractice in which people have posed as fertility specialists and 'treated' unwitting patients at great expense. Given a widespread lack of medical knowledge within the community and deference to authority figures, such fraudulent cases spread misgivings about seeking treatment. For example, Ladda experienced a lack of appropriate referrals and iatrogenic treatment which delayed her quest for infertility treatment. Her vulnerability was compounded by her lack of familiarity with the medical profession and poor communication. Ladda sought treatment after she failed to fall pregnant for five years following her marriage. When she was thirty years old Ladda sought medical care but did not know whom to see. Following a friend's advice she went to see a doctor although she did not realize at the time that, although a gynaecologist, the doctor did not have much expertise with infertility:

> The doctor was a family planning doctor. There was no medical equipment or anything. I had a physical examination, blood examination and many other examinations, and then the clinic gave me paperwork to get an x-ray done in *Pratu Nam* [Watergate]. I rarely visited a doctor because I hardly got sick so I had no idea what to expect. I went to a place where I was supposed to get an x-ray done. I did not get any x-ray dye injection. They inserted equipment to my womb and turned it back and forth. The doctor, who did the x-ray for me, wondered why I decided to see this [family planning] doctor. I was curious why the doctor asked me this strange question but the [x-ray] doctor did not say much. I got paranoid but still went back there even though I had no idea what they would do to me.... The clinic gave me some medications to help me ovulate. They still did not explain to me much. I did not quite understand why I had to have the medications but when I asked the doctor, he still did not say much. After taking the medication, I went in to get an injection [IUI], then I was pushed out [in a cart] from a delivery room to another recovery room. There were so many people staring at me as if I just came out from an abortion. I was so embarrassed.... It did not work then so I

> never went back there again. It was my first time and I had no idea what they did to me. I was so embarrassed and did not go back there for about a year. I don't know if it was my body itself, the medication or the x-ray but I lost all of my hair. I did not know what to do so I went back to the same doctor. I told the doctor that I did not have a period for about three months and lost all my hair. He thought that the reason I had not come back to him was because I got pregnant. I had blood, urine examination et cetera and found out that I was not pregnant. He gave me some antihistamine but it still did not help. I was so worried. I went in and out of clinics so often as if I was there for shopping.... Doctors did not say anything. We are just ordinary people and we have no idea.... Once I stopped the medications, the symptoms had gone and I had my hair back again.

After a two-year delay because of this incident Ladda read about assisted reproduction in a book and so decided to attend that doctor's clinic. At that clinic it was discovered that she had a tumour that was blocking one of her fallopian tubes. She underwent surgery. After moving to another hospital she discovered that the original surgery had failed to remove the tumour. She required further endoscopic surgery in which the affected tube was totally removed.

> It's possible that they [at the first hospital] made a mistake and found that there was nothing inside [during the first surgery] so they sew it back. I was thinking about going back to Dr T but I was told that perhaps it was my luck that they did not take the whole uterus out. If so, I would not be here right now [for fertility treatment]. Though, I am still not happy with Dr T that he lied. The doctor here [at this hospital] could see that I was ripped off from Dr T before so they did not charge me a fortune. They also gave me a videotape for an evidence of what they had had taken out.

Nuchnari and Somkhit were being treated in a leading private clinic that specializes in infertility. They moved after being told Nuchnari would require surgery to remove fibroids removed at another private hospital. They sought a second opinion:

> With the P [private] Hospital, they diagnosed that my wife had fascia/fibroids and that they needed to be removed first. When we told the doctor here [at this clinic], he told us that he could not see the need for such surgery after the diagnosis. The doctor at the P [private] Hospital told us that my wife could not be pregnant unless she got the fascia/fibroids removed. We also needed to have around forty to fifty thousand baht (US $1,300–$1,450) ready for the surgery. We do not have a problem with such amount of money but my sister had had such surgery before and she had to recuperate for months. She could

> not work strenuously. Besides, there are no guarantees that my wife would be able to get pregnant. We were so shocked after hearing from the doctor here that we did not need such surgery. It would be like we hurt ourselves for nothing if we decided to go through with the surgery. That's why I am so impressed with this clinic.

Such cases of a lack of transparency in treatment may be the result of poor communication or poor practice but also reveal how the image of a doctor as that of a healer with special moral status and expertise may transform into an image of a doctor as a businessman engaged in profit-making activity. The experience of what is believed to be profit gouging or over-servicing leaves patients suspicious of the practice of medicine and the character and motivations of physicians. They stand in contrast to the continued portrayal of doctors as beneficent and virtuous and the practice of healing and medicine as a form of merit making. Accusations of profiteering can be especially acute in assisted reproduction when the costs are so high and results unreliable.

Conclusions

In Thailand healing has always been regarded as a noble calling and imbued with religious merit. Doctors occupy a high status in Thai society, a status further enhanced by the high-tech science of reproductive medicine – markers of modernity and progress. As seen in chapter 1, media renditions of reproductive specialists have projected an image of 'men of science' capable of miracle feats, giving and sustaining life. In this chapter staff working the field of reproductive medicine describe themselves as undertaking a special vocation to assist the infertile; some have personal experience of infertility. Yet the care they extend to their patients in their portrayals of themselves is not always perceived in the same way. Patients generally adopt an attitude of respectful submission to their doctors, working with the clinical ensemble towards achievement of a pregnancy. Yet their lack of questions often leaves them lacking answers, communication can be minimal or poorly understood and what is an everyday matter for clinic staff can be a new, unsettling and embarrassing experience for patients. But most Thai patients will be reluctant to publically criticize their doctor or question his/her judgement. If they have a successful pregnancy patients may describe their doctors as quasi-divine. However, as in their interactions with other divine beings, for patients the outcomes may be fickle and uncertain. The failure of a cycle makes both patient and doctor lose face: the patient is reminded of the imperfections of his or her body or a failure to follow recommended lifestyle, rest or drug regimens or poor karma; a doctor stands vulnerable to accusations of a lack of expertise or profiteering. The technologies themselves are rarely questioned. With the chances of failure so high, the relationships between patients and their doctors often become strained and patients move to seek care elsewhere and undergo further interventions until they gradually become cynical about the claims and promises offered by the medical profession.

Chapter 6

Patriarchal Bargains

Gender identities and relations are deeply enmeshed in the use and practices of assisted reproduction. Use of these technologies makes visible one's status as infertile. Not only are assisted reproductive technologies themselves gendered in their specific and differentiated application to women and men's bodies (Konrad 1998), but they have profound effects upon women and men's relationships and notions of femininity and masculinity. Thompson (2005) notes how normative repertoires of femininity, masculinity, fatherhood and motherhood are evoked to justify, applaud and stabilize gender identities of infertile couples and the interventions of technology into reproduction.

As described in chapter 4, women's bodies are the sites for most interventions during treatment. Feminist scholarship has questioned the value and effects of new reproductive technologies and whether they diminish or enhance women's power over reproduction in the process (Becker 2000; Birke, Himmelweit and Vines 1990; Franklin 1990; Rapp 1990, 1999; Sandelowski 1990, 1991). Current studies now present more nuanced considerations of the complexity of actors, interests, agency and outcomes (see review by Thompson 2002).

Infertility and its treatment affect the dynamics of couples' relationships and marriages. The stress of treatment regimes, feelings of guilt and loss and interventions into couples' sexual lives all take a toll on their relationships. But the very presence of the options offered by assisted reproductive technologies may introduce 'motherhood mandates' (Thompson 2002) – added pressures particularly upon women who may feel obliged or pressured to try these technologies. Marcia Inhorn's (1996) work among Egyptian women maps the exhaustive struggles of women to achieve motherhood in a highly patriarchal society where men are permitted to pursue divorce if their wives fail to produce a child. In Egypt infertility carries heavy stigma within a patriarchal society in which the ability to bear children is a source of power for women. She explores the broad context of Middle Eastern gender politics, and the ways in which this articulates with religious and class membership to mediate the experience of women. Her work reveals the extraordinary lengths to which couples will go to avail themselves of the costly procedures. Poor women carry a triple stigma due to their gender, poverty and inability to bear children. They are blamed for their failure to produce children and undergo therapeutic quests that can be 'traumatic and often unfruitful' (Inhorn 1994: 3).

Marcia Inhorn (1996, 2003) describes how infertility may have a range of consequences for conjugal relationships in Egypt. As she notes (2003a: 222), there has been relatively little research situating the experience of IVF and infertility for women *'as lived with their husbands'* (emphasis in original). In some cases feelings of conjugal connectivity may be strengthened by the absence of children, but for other couples the experience and treatment of infertility provokes a crisis of commitment. The advent of technologies such as ICSI has had direct implications for some Egyptian marriages as men choose between older first wives and younger and more fertile women to improve their chances of success (Inhorn 2002, 2003a). For men, too, tensions may arise if they are the infertile partner, an issue I explore further in chapter 8.

This chapter contributes to understanding how Thai women utilize and frame the use of assisted reproductive technologies according to local understandings of gender relations, womanhood, marriage and reproduction. I argue that to understand why women undergo the arduous process of IVF treatment it is necessary to understand the importance of reproduction to conjugal and family relationships. It is also important to understand women's own expectations of how having children will change their lives and relationships.

As noted in chapter 2 in Thailand children are understood to bind the relationship of a married couple together and ensure the continuation of the family line across generations. The failure to produce a child within the first few years of married life brings questions from in-laws and friends and exposes the intimate politics within women's relationships with their husbands, their families and society.

Apart from their own desires for affirmation and fulfilment through having children, Thai women in this study express a desire to overcome their infertility as a means of forming and consolidating their relationship with their spouse. Although it can be argued that the Thai women who appear in the following pages are not as constrained as their Egyptian counterparts, in Thailand, women describe an ever-present fear of divorce or their husbands' finding a *mia noi*, or 'minor wife', if they fail to satisfy his desires for a child. Their involvement in IVF is often mixed with fears regarding the consequences for their family life if they are not successful.

This chapter presents two case studies. The first examines Pook's fears of her husband deserting her if assisted reproduction fails. Her case illustrates how for some women involvement in IVF is a strategic and pragmatic act to secure their relationships. The second case study of Nut and her husband Manit can be read in multiple ways. One reading is of a relationship that has been strengthened through the use of assisted reproduction. But it also provides an example where the regime of care enforced by the husband asserts patriarchal male control, restricting Nut in the name of ensuring the success of the treatment. I argue that both cases represent forms of 'patriarchal bargaining' through which women secure their relationships.

The broader issue addressed by this chapter is the ongoing debate on whether these technologies enhance women's reproductive choice or facilitate oppression by men and the medical profession (for example, see Corea 1988; Pfeffer 1993; Rothman 1989). At the core of this debate lies fundamental anthropological concerns regarding the nature of agency within conditions of gendered, class and racial inequality. Heather Paxson (2003: 1858) notes that many earlier studies of assisted reproduction depict it as something women submit to. She offers a more nuanced view of the agency of women in using these technologies. Greek women speak of assisted reproduction as something women 'do' and achieve rather than submit to. She suggests that assisted reproductive technologies are viewed in Greece as woman-centred procedures and Greek women are granted considerable reproductive agency and practical control over using these technologies, although they do so within the confines of patriarchal family relations. She notes 'women's reproductive agency can emerge in ways that simultaneously reformat and reproduce social relations, including patriarchal inequalities' (Paxson 2003: 1864). In this chapter I explore how utilization of assisted reproduction in Thailand occurs within patriarchal family relations and involves actions that simultaneously may redefine and reproduce patriarchal inequalities.

Fear of Marriage Instability

Fear of future instability in marriage was an important motivation for many women to seek care. Instability was particularly feared among couples where only one partner was infertile. In particular, infertile women feared that their husbands would have extramarital affairs or support a *mia noi*, or divorce them if they failed to produce a child. This fear and expectation of Thai men's infidelity is not isolated to couples with fertility difficulties, but is a common finding in studies of Thai marriage (Packard-Winkler 1996; Saengtienchai et al. 1999). However, it is acute for women who perceive themselves as having failed to fulfil their husband's expectations of marriage by failing to produce a child. Lek was worried that 'if nothing comes to knit the relationship together then I'm afraid the family will fall apart so I decided to come and see a doctor.... Normally our relationship is good but now here it has improved a little. We are more concerned about each other.' Tuk said she was undergoing treatment 'because I am afraid of future problems.... If we don't have a child in the future my husband may have another woman. Because he hasn't got a [fertility] problem. We don't know the future.' Ton observed, 'From some couples I have seen, [if the treatment isn't successful] the husband would have a mistress because he really wants to have a baby.' In some cases men place pressure upon their wives to undergo treatment. For example, Pui was just starting treatment and described how she was very scared of injections and the pain of IVF but was undergoing treatment to please her husband. She suggested her act was a form of 'gift' for her husband that demonstrated her commitment to him: 'He said we should try. If it [a pregnancy] doesn't stick we'll keep doing it until it succeeds however many times it takes ... he really wants to have a baby.... Because I am scared. I'm afraid that it might hurt. [But] my husband, he begged me. So I came. He said, "Whatever [happens] we have to do it anyway." So I came.'

Women who had been previously divorced felt added pressure to consolidate their second relationships through children. Laiat is in her second marriage. She had two children from her first marriage, a ten-year-old boy and a twelve-year-old girl. She tearfully related how her first husband, a lawyer, prevents her from having any contact with them:

> My ex-husband is giving me a hard time. I don't know the reason. The thing is I endowed everything to my children. He is a lawyer and wants to be their guardian. I found out later that he had sold the house we bought together without my permission. I don't know where they are. He moved the children to another school.... I am not sure if he's taken them to Choomporn. I went to see them at their school once; the little one was only five, he could not recognize me, the older one is very scared of her new parents. They perhaps threaten them not to see me. He hit me and would not let me see them.... Now, I don't even know where they are.

As is common practice among women in Thailand, Laiat had a tubal ligation following the birth of her second child. She has had it reversed in her attempt to give her new husband a child of his own.

> I told him before we got married [that I was sterilized] and never kept it a secret because I want him to accept who I am. I am divorced and it is not so acceptable in Thai society. At the beginning, my husband was nervous to tell his mother that he was with me. Once I see them more often and feel closer to each other, they are so wonderful to me. I told them that I was sterilized and the chance of having a child was almost a zero. I was honest with them that I could have the reversal of tubal ligation earlier but I did not want to fall pregnant before we got married. His mother is a real conservative Chinese, there will be so much pressure for me if we cannot have a baby. However, she might come to terms with not having a grandchild as her son [my husband] almost did not get married because he is already fifty years old. She perhaps did not think that he would ever get married. I have asked him before why he did not look for a younger girl so that she could give him a baby. It must be destiny that brought us together.

As for many of the women in this study, for Laiat the use of assisted reproductive technologies is both a means of fulfilling maternal desires, and a pragmatic act to secure her relationships and demonstrate her commitment to her husband and her in-laws. The case study of Pook below illustrates the insecurity behind many women's treatment seeking.

Pook: 'If I Had a Choice I Wouldn't Do It'

Pook was in the clinic waiting for an ultrasound to see how many eggs she had produced after stimulation. She was thin and looked exhausted. She was trying her first cycle of IVF at a public hospital. Pook has one fifteen-year-old son from a previous marriage who usually lives with his grandparents in Khorat in Northeast Thailand for his schooling. Now thirty-five years old she has been married to her current husband ten years.

> It was easy for me to have a baby with my first husband but with my second husband we have been married for ten years but haven't fallen pregnant so we wondered why. After five years we started seeing a doctor in Khorat but we didn't succeed. We didn't have continuous treatment because we kept moving so when we settled in Suphan permanently then I came here to have treatment.

Pook was feeling very discouraged and tired after a long trip from her orchard farm in a neighbouring province to attend the clinic. She had woken before sunrise and travelled several hours by motorcycle taxi, then a two-bench truck (*songthaew*), then a van and finally river ferry to get to the hospital. She usually comes alone as her husband 'doesn't want to come' and some weeks she has appointments three days a week. As orchardists she and her husband are not particularly wealthy. They wanted to start treatment when she was still in her twenties but needed to save money, so only now can they afford the treatment:

> The treatment costs a lot of money so we have to save a lot of money. It is very discouraging. I don't know whether it is going to stick or not. We have to spend all of our savings just for this because we don't have a career that can generate us a lot of money. The treatment has a high cost. If we are successful I'll be happy but at the moment I am starting to feel discouraged. Every time I come here there is always a problem.

After painful surgical investigations she has been told she has two blocked fallopian tubes while her husband is normal. She thinks an injection after the birth of her first child is responsible for her secondary infertility. She had been told she had an infection in her uterus (*mot luk aksep,* มดลูกอักเสบ).

> A month after the birth of the first baby I had an infection in the womb so I had an injection and since then I haven't fallen pregnant even though [in the past] I could have a baby easily. But after I had an injection from that clinic they [pregnancies] didn't stick at all. I don't know what they injected into me. I haven't taken any [contraceptive] tablets or had any [Depo provera] injections for ten years.

Although she already has a child from her previous relationship, Pook is undertaking IVF treatment in the hope that it will improve and consolidate her new relationship: 'I think it will improve [our relationship]. It will make the family complete. I have my own baby [from a previous relationship] but my husband hasn't [had a child]. If he has his own he will be complete and maybe won't want to go anywhere [to have extramarital relationships]. Maybe he will stay with the family. Help each other. At the moment it is not complete.'

Her husband puts pressure on her to come for treatment: 'He wants to have a child very much. He's wanted one since when we were first married. We didn't use contraception from the start. He is stressed that we haven't had one, because he had an examination with the doctor and his sperm is strong. He loves kids very much so he puts pressure on me.' The pressure has included threats to find another woman.

> Every time we talk about it we have a problem about it [arguing]. He said that he would go and get a *mia noi* if I don't have a baby, so I must try. I am afraid that there will be problems in our family. He wants to have his own baby. I have already got a child, I don't want to have anymore. It's difficult for me to have another so I don't want to have another. I don't know whether he is serious or just joking about (the *mia noi*). But when he said this it made me upset. His semen is good. If he went with another person, a new wife he could have a baby straight away. So I must try no matter how painful it is, I must bear it. I'm afraid that my husband might have a new wife.

She also feels pressure from her husband's family to bear them a child. They are encouraging their son to find a new wife if she is unable to bear him one: 'They put pressure on me in every way. Whatever pain is involved I must bear it. Do whatever I have to do. His siblings all have kids. So he wants his own child. [There is] a lot of pressure. Sometimes I think a lot. Why do others have babies easily? Why do I have to spend a lot of money on this? He puts a lot of pressure on me.'

She is using up all her savings to undertake the treatment and only has enough money to do IVF two or possibly three times.

> My friends don't know about this. I haven't told anyone, I don't want to tell anyone. I am doing this quietly. Just in case it is not successful I am afraid they might criticize me saying I wasted money for nothing. I have only this much income but still went and did it. So I don't want to tell anyone. It is only known within the family. If my friends ask me where I have been I say I've been to see a doctor. If it is successful then I will tell them but at this moment I am scared to tell them.

Pook admitted that she didn't want to undertake IVF but needed to do it to satisfy her husband's wishes:

> No. I don't want to do it. It is very tiring, painful, wastes my time when I could work and earn. If I could choose I wouldn't do it. If I had a choice I wouldn't do it. I wouldn't come. I'm doing this because of pressure; I am not that desperate for a baby.... But my husband said I must do it otherwise he will have another wife. If I try to the max he might have sympathy with me. If I don't try he won't sympathise with me and will find a new wife straight away. [If he did] he'll have a child straight away as his sperm is very strong. Although he is forty he's still strong. All the pressure is on me. Sometimes I am so stressed I don't sleep at all. At night I am stressed. Before I came here [to the clinic] I was stressed. After I came and knew what the problem was I was stressed. I returned home and thought a lot and I don't sleep.... He has power. He is the one who works. I don't work as hard as he does. I have to do whatever he says. If I don't then we fight. There is always a problem. Because what he says goes. I must follow him. If I don't there will be a problem. He gets upset with me and peeved with me and won't come home. So I stay at home alone. Every time we fight or have problems he goes to his relatives place and I'm by myself.

Ten days later we met Pook again at the clinic. She was about to have embryos transferred. The ova extraction had been very painful for her and she spent three days in considerable pain unable to walk with no one around to help her. She wasn't sure how many eggs had been retrieved:

> I wanted to ask the doctor exactly how many eggs I got but the doctor left before I could. I asked my friend how many eggs she got and she said over ten and the other patients who had eggs collected on that day got seven to eight. I think I got four eggs. Very few. If I do it and they don't stick then I have to start again and waste more money. Rich people have so many eggs, people with no money trying their best and get very few eggs. But I have to ask the doctor again. [During the extraction] I heard everything and I felt the doctor stir something in my vagina I felt that I would like the doctor to finish the egg collection quickly. It hurt.

Her husband had not accompanied her to the transfer and she planned to return by public transport again to her home to rest. 'I must rest. If I don't have a rest I can't stand it. Otherwise, if my body is not good, it [the embryo] won't stick ... I won't do anything. Even if he asks me to I won't. I'll tell him that I can't, I have a pain in the stomach. Even if he tells me to I won't. Let him do it. This is very difficult. I am by myself. When I am in pain no one looks after me. Very, very hard.' Pook was deeply concerned that she might use all her savings on IVF to no avail and that her husband would abandon her, leaving her and her son with no financial support and no assets. She felt obliged to at least try IVF so she could be seen to have tried her best to produce him a child: 'If I have tried this much and still have a problem then I can't stand it. If I didn't try then he might have a reason to criticize me. But now that I am trying if it doesn't stick whatever happens, so be it.'

We followed up with a phone call to Pook three months later. On that cycle only five eggs had been retrieved of which only two were suitable. They transferred two embryos but without success. Pook was taking a break from further treatment as she had used up all her savings and so needed to work and save more money. She intended undergoing another cycle in the future.

For women such as Pook, the very existence of assisted reproductive technologies means she is expected to try everything possible to satisfy her husband's desire for a child, despite the fact that she does not particularly want another child. Much is at stake if her latest marriage fails. Although recently reformed, in the past Thai family law discriminated heavily against women and stories of women losing custody of children and being left with no property or assets following a divorce are rife. She is not financially independent. There remains little protection for women should divorce settlements not be honoured.

Pook's and Laiat's cases highlight a latent threat articulated by many women in the study: the fear of ending up both childless and without a partner. Having fully subscribed to Thai ideals of motherhood and family, contemplating the future without these evokes a crisis of meaning and makes each unsuccessful cycle and setback more stressful. Added to this is the background pressure from family members – in particular parents-in-law to produce a grandchild – who sometimes counsel divorce or threaten disinheritance should an heir not be produced. Under such circumstances women may find themselves subject to pressure from the older generation of women in the family. Women with no children have little power within family relationships and some reported constant questions and monitoring from their mothers-in-law about whether they were pregnant. In chapter 2, for example, I noted that Ploy stated the only reason she was undergoing IVF was 'because my mother-in-law really wants to have a grandchild. Whenever we go to visit her, she would complain that she felt embarrassed that she still does not have any grandchildren.... She kept asking me when I would get treatment.' Her own mother was opposed to her treatment.

Effects of Treatment on Relationships

Women and men have different experiences of assisted reproduction (Greil, Leitko and Porter 1988). As a number of authors have noted, women often bear the brunt of the medical interventions, even when male infertility factors are the cause of their inability to have a child. This can produce tensions in the relationship. Mai commented that she did not feel her husband fully appreciated the pain and burden that undergoing treatment involved for her: 'Only collecting semen for him. He did not need to go through what I had been through every day; no need to get injections, no need to worry about taking medication on time, no need to insert the hormones into him.' A source of tension can arise if a partner is not felt to be equally committed to treatment. For example, Ploy complained: 'I feel that I have been trying so hard and I want my husband to cut down on his alcohol consumption even if he is under stress. I want everything to be ready. I have quit my job to work at home, I am ready. On one occasion, he still drank before we came here for the IUI appointment [which can affect the quality of the sperm produced]. I was so disappointed about it.' The need to have regular sexual relations at times determined by the treatment also caused strain to her relationship with her husband:

> Part of the problem might be that we are not intimate so often.... My husband is stressed. He brings work home. He feels tired and just wants to sleep. He loses his mood if the air conditioning is not cold enough. Even after the hormonal injections we could not do it [have sex] as often as the doctor told us. I think he is the problem because my physical examination is normal. But my husband does not agree. He thinks I am the one [who is infertile] because I often get sick.

As in the case of Ploy, a number of the women in this study had given up their work to pursue treatment with an assumption they would soon be pregnant and unable to work anyway, a common pattern in Thailand where few jobs carry any maternity benefits. Giving up paid employment shifted the power relations in their marriages, making them financially and socially more dependent upon their husbands. Although women spoke of the benefits of giving up work which allowed them to freely attend treatment appointments, rest when required, avoid stress and tiring commuting, they also saw this as another sacrifice undertaken for treatment, a fundamental change to their financial independence but also their identity.

Although fears of marital instability were common, as noted above, some couples stated that their relationships had been strengthened by their experience of undergoing IVF treatment. Mai noted the enormous pressure that treatment placed upon her relationship with her husband, but noted that through the hardship of treatment she had come to appreciate the support her husband gave:

> The problem was that it put a lot pressure on our emotions and relationship. Sometimes, it led to arguments with no reasons. I was very disappointed with the whole thing so I wanted to take a break for about two months before I came back for the third time.... My husband was very good to me. He was very understanding and provided me with good moral support. When I got angry and frustrated, he would keep quiet.... Even when I was irritable, he would keep quiet. I could see that he was also upset but he did not want to show me [his true feeling]. We would comfort each other that it was not our fault. We told ourselves that we not only needed a good doctor, but we also needed good timing and good luck on our sides. We had to talk and support each other. My husband was always there for me. Some people, who have no problem with infertility, would not understand.

Similarly, Mot declared that while undergoing treatment, 'he took better care of me. Especially during the IUI treatment, I did not need to do anything. He would do everything for me'. Porn and Aruth was one of the few couples to openly speak of love (*khwamrak*) when talking about their relationship and spoke of the increased understanding and improved communication that had resulted from their experience of treatment: 'We love each other even more (since the treatment). We talk more. If there is a problem we support each other more.' They had come to realize that they could live contentedly together even if no child results from their treatment.

Nut and Manit

At one level the case of Nut and Manit is a success story as they were fortunate to be pregnant with a son after their first cycle of IVF-ICSI at a private hospital. They have been married for three years and decided to investigate their fertility after about two years when they had not fallen pregnant. Nut was found to have a small growth in her uterus and Manit had a low sperm count. Previous IUI treatment at another hospital had been unsuccessful so they had decided to undergo IVF-ICSI. When we first met them at their private hospital they were undergoing prenatal genetic tests on the pregnancy, checking for Down's syndrome and other genetic problems. They described themselves as 'happy, very happy, extremely happy' about the pregnancy. A well-dressed, attractive couple, Nut is thirty-six years old and had an undergraduate education and had given up her job with a company to undergo IVF and her husband is a forty-six years' old legal specialist with postgraduate qualifications. The couple was interviewed together, Manit dominating the discussion.

They wanted to provide an heir and grandchild for their parents, but also saw having a family as making their family complete. As noted in chapter 2, Manit described children as a 'golden chain' linking parents, and as an affirmation of their responsibility, maturity and marriage: 'If you don't have babies, if you don't have grandchildren, what are you going to do? It's not that we want a baby so that they can look after us, it is because we want to have a companion for the mother and look after our assets. People with families have responsibilities, a house and assets … to fulfil your life.'

After the ICSI procedure they had five 'beautiful' embryos ready for transfer. Two were frozen for later use. The initial attempt to transfer the embryos failed and was very painful because of problems with her fallopian tubes which required expansion. They were shocked at this setback but 'part of me was thinking that, OK it isn't the right auspicious time for the baby to be born. The baby isn't ready to be born. As Buddhists, we believe people have their auspicious time to be born and to die.' As noted in chapter 2, this appeal to the Buddhist notion of the child not being ready to be born and the need for the timing to be correct allowed them to appeal to the mysteries of the spiritual world for responsibility for the failure of their IVF cycle. Such a view complicates the procreative agency involved in IVF: the notion of fertility as a technical problem with a technical solution and IVF doctors as instrumental in the success of couples. Ultimately, according to this philosophy, human intervention is undertaken, but the success or failure of the intervention depends on karma and the fate of the mother and child.

Following the next attempt to transfer the blastocysts, Nut was driven to her mother's home in another province to rest for two weeks before undergoing a pregnancy test. Once the pregnancy was confirmed, Nut submitted herself to a regime of rest and seclusion under the care of her husband. She initially took leave from work but once her pregnancy was confirmed, her husband insisted she quit her job to avoid getting tired: '[I have to] stay home only, doing nothing till I deliver the baby.'

Manit attributed their successful pregnancy to this period of confined rest: 'What I notice is that the treatment fails because the mother works. Just having days off on weekend is not enough. Taking leave for two weeks after the embryo transfer is not enough. It has to be at least two months.' Nut described that period of rest: '[I] couldn't do anything, couldn't walk, just eat and sleep. For almost two months. It's a two storey house and I stayed upstairs and wasn't allowed to go out of my bedroom. I could just stay in my bedroom for two months.' She was monitored closely by her husband throughout this time. He described the regime:

> I cooked and then brought food to her upstairs. After she finished eating, I would take her plates to wash. I did all the housework including looking after our dogs. Normally we share the housework. It's not too much to ask. [Men] should be understanding and make sacrifice. It's because women have to tolerate more than men. Their body/anatomy is more complicated than that of a man, especially when they have a baby in their tummy. So we men should be understanding. ... The better we look after our wife, the baby will also [receive that care]. If her mental state isn't good it will flow onto the baby because they are connected.... So, what I did, it's not that I did it for nothing. Housework is nothing [compared to my work]. It [housework] is nothing. That's why I say, if you are serious [about doing IVF] you have to understand each other very much and love each other fondly. You have to make sacrifice. You have to do things you have never done before. And this also applies to your wife. What you used to do you have to stop doing. It's not that you can't tolerate not doing what you want to do, you have to control yourself, you can't be like you used to.

Nut commented: 'I have never felt that there would be any man who can look after a woman. Seriously! As far as I know, there is no man who can look after a woman this well. And that man happens to look after me. He stopped me from doing anything. After I eat, I stay in my room. I am almost able to count how many steps I took.'

Despite her appreciation of his care, the surveillance and control of her activities was oppressive. She only was allowed to 'watch movies, listen to music, play games, eat and then sleep'.

> Nut: During those two months that I did nothing, I was stressed. When I was stressed I was grumpy. I wanted to do this, do that. Could I do them?
>
> Manit: [She] wanted to go shopping.
>
> Nut: No. I wanted to do some light housework.

> Manit: I had to scold her. Sometimes when you talk nicely then they won't listen to you so you have to rouse on them. Right? In your life, how many years have you spent shopping? You just have to bear this [not shopping] for another one or two months then you can shop any time.

In this exchange he belittled her desire to do something around the house, claiming it was merely a frivolous feminine desire to shop. The onus of responsibility of success was totally placed on Nut, whose movement and tasks were completely restricted for a number of months. In this she submitted to control by her husband but came to resent his insistence that she stop all work and not do anything. Avoidance of any chance of 'an accident' that could jeopardize the precious pregnancy became the priority. Her status as a potential mother, a carrier of an embryo, subsumed all else.

Both Nut and Manit said that their experience of IVF had strengthened their relationship. In particular, the inversion of roles within the home, with Manit undertaking most of the housework, was cited as particularly significant. Nut commented: 'I can see positive effects. I can see more happiness and bonds. But since the first day we started the treatment, he has changed and looked after me like … before I looked after him, I was doing my housewife duties and he was a husband. After I got the embryo transfer, he became both housewife and house husband. He did everything.' Manit stated that the experience had given him greater understanding of women's suffering during pregnancy:

> Sometimes, you know, guys are used to being looked after all the time. When it's my turn to do this, it makes me realize that it's not easy for my wife to do this either [to look after a husband]. If the guy could get pregnant, they would know that it hurts/is painful for women and women have to endure it. It's not like that, I have to do it [look after her]. It's not compulsory or anything. It's hard for her to look after me. It's like when you get married she looks after her husband everyday and the husband just waits at the table shaking his leg and waiting when the food will be served. Now if the husband returns that for the wife, the husband will realize that, mmm, my wife has to put up with a lot.

Nut responded: 'I think that it is the responsibility that we have to look after the husband. But I think what he is doing is not his responsibility but he is doing it anyway. And he is doing it in excess of what I want.'

Manit claimed that the experience of IVF had given him greater insight into his wife. However, undergoing IVF had reinforced a firmly patriarchal relationship between Nut and Manit in which he took over control of nearly all aspects of her life during the pregnancy. Although the gendered division of housework was inverted, there is a fine line between 'care' and 'control'. Experience of IVF had 'strengthened' their relationship but the onus of responsibility of success was placed on Nut. She completely restricted her movement and tasks for a number of months. Although she submitted to the regime imposed by her husband, it is clear that at times she resented the degree to which he policed her activities. Her status as a potential mother, carrier of an embryo, subsumed all else. Once pregnant, Nut was constructed as incapable of doing even minor work around the house, her body a fragile vessel for the baby that needed monitoring and discipline. She was ordered to stop working. Any resistance on her part was viewed as irresponsibly threatening the future child. At a later interview three months later when reflecting upon their experience, Manit said:

> The hardest thing was when I asked her to stop working and she didn't want to, she still wanted to work. Secondly, it's when I had to work and she stayed home, I was afraid that she mightn't be able to cope. And then do things that she was not supposed to do like walking down [the stairs], cleaning the house, cleaning the floor. That's beyond my ability to see because I had to work. She was at home alone and I was worried whether she would be able to bear this. Would she do things that I told her not to do? That was my worry.

For Nut, submission to Manit's discipline was difficult: 'One month is already bad enough to do nothing and this was three months [staying in my bedroom]. Three months made my mind/spirit terrible. But with his consolation, threatening, scolding, all [that] helped me get through because I have him by my side. He did everything for us, for baby, thinking back, things that he has done are the best things for us but back then I didn't appreciate it.'

At a telephone interview in January the couple were excited, as the baby was due to be born through an elective caesarean section. Later that month Nut gave birth to a healthy son. They intended to tell their child of his conception through a diary and photograph album, 'this is the start of your life from when the sperm was injected ... it was so hard for your parents to have you and this is what we want him to know'.

Conclusions: Agency and Patriarchal Bargains in Assisted Reproduction

Many of the women in this study described consenting to assisted reproductive treatment to maintain their relationships and strengthen their position within families as much as to fulfil their own personal desires to experience pregnancy and nurture a child. In doing so they may be prepared to undergo painful interventions, give up paid employment, submit to the control of their husband and the medical profession and risk their financial security. A number of early radical feminist writings on IVF suggested that women's consent to undergo treatment was not a true choice, given societal pressures upon women to reproduce (see, for example, Corea et al. 1987; Rothman 1989). But such characterizations of women denies their agency. Jodi Jacobson (2000: 26) suggests that across the reproductive health literature such representations 'fail to give women their due as autonomous agents and turn them into dupes and victims by suggesting that their choices are but mindless capitulations of social pressures'. Deniz Kandiyoti has argued for a more nuanced consideration of the constant negotiations women undergo in their relationships with male dominated institutions and patriarchy: 'Women strategize within a set of concrete constraints that reveal and define the blueprint of ... the *patriarchal bargain* of any given society' (1991: 104, emphasis in original). She suggests that women's personal and political struggles are often complex and at times contradictory and may include instances where women collude with increased control by men. This would include instances described above, such as undergoing IVF to attempt to ensure the financial and social security of a marriage for oneself and one's child (as in the case of Pook) or giving up paid employment and submitting to a restrictive regime controlled by one's husband (as in the case of Nut) in return for his admiration, a secure relationship and a much desired child. Kandiyoti (1991: 114) suggests that such patriarchal bargains 'do not merely inform women's rational choices but also shape the more unconscious aspects of their gendered subjectivity, because they permeate the context of their early socialization, as well as their adult cultural milieu'. In this case these strategies are undertaken in the context of several levels of constraints including; the unequal status of women in most Thai heterosexual relationships, the moral imperative that women should be mothers, the emphasis upon 'bloodlines' and biological inheritance, an ideology of male sexual privilege, differing expectations of fidelity in marriage and the belief that children make a relationship and individual 'complete'. Above all is the fact that in Thai society the social burden of childlessness and the burden of its treatment continues to fall disproportionately upon women. Failure to produce a child risks exposure to social and economic insecurity. Women make decisions about undergoing assisted reproductive treatment within this context. They make pragmatic decisions within particular cultural and structural settings and it is the nature of these social and material conditions under which choices are made that is the critical issue. As could be expected of this sample from people already undergoing treatment at clinics, most women in this study were committed to their decision to undergo treatment. As evident from their accounts in chapter 4, their agency and desire for a child with their partner should not be dismissed. However, it is particularly disturbing to find women such as Pook who frankly stated that they were undergoing treatment not out of their own desire for a child, but to please their husbands and secure their relationships, and that the doctors treating them in some cases hadn't bothered to ask about their circumstances.

This also draws attention to the ways in which notions of women's agency behind earlier feminist studies of IVF assume a Western notion of individuality that is not necessarily unproblematic in Asian societies. The emphasis on individual autonomy assumed in these studies ignores the significant family, cultural and social relationships and collective identities in many cultural settings. In Thai and Sino-Thai families in particular, one's status as a member of a family line or kin group may have great influence over individual decision making. A woman's decisions over treatment involves more than concerns over her bodily well-being, but also displays of filial duty, maintenance of social status and intergenerational continuity.

Utilizing IVF challenges normative frameworks of meaning surrounding reproduction in Thailand, subverting ideas of 'natural' reproductive processes and kinship and positing new ways in which maternity and paternity may be experienced. Yet at the same time it is used to ratify social ideas surrounding gender norms and maintain unequal power relations between women and men, and submission to the medicalization of their bodies. Women resort to assisted reproductive treatments with varying degrees of enthusiasm and for differing reasons. As demonstrated in the previous chapter, many women are more than willing participants, but as described in this chapter, others speak with ambivalence and resentment over the choices they have made or the lack of choices they experience. For some, reproductive treatment becomes a time when they become most keenly aware of their unequal position and status as women, and the power relations in their relationships with their husbands and families. Their search for support is described in the following chapter.

Judith Lorber (1989) suggests that although women's desires to undergo treatment when they themselves are infertile are understandable, less understandable is the consent of women to undergo treatment to enable an infertile male partner to father a child. As will be discussed in chapter 8, a number of women whose partners were infertile described undergoing IVF-ICSI procedures on their otherwise healthy fertile bodies to 'please' their husbands because their husbands were 'good' men with whom they wished to have a child. Such decisions are represented by women as 'gifts' to their husbands, demonstrations of their love and commitment to the relationship, but must also be read within the gendered expectations described above, whereby it is assumed that the treatment of infertility is not just about an individual woman's body, but a couple, family and intergenerational concern. But men too are involved in 'patriarchal bargains' as they attempt to fulfil social expectations of Thai masculinity and paternity and chapter 8 considers the experience of treatment by men and considers how they negotiate the use of these technologies.

Notes

1. *Mot luk aksep*, literally an inflamed or infected uterus, is an ambiguous term used for a range of reproductive tract infections and conditions by medical personnel and by lay people. It is also used as a translation for pelvic inflammatory disease. It is interesting that here she blames the treatment of an infection rather than the infection for the damage to her reproductive tract.

Chapter 7

'Love Clinic'

Online Communities

> This is the first time I have written here but in the past I have been reading with all my friends and have learned a lot and my confidence has increased now I know that I am not alone with this problem. – Kitty, 27 January 2007

> I am sending you strength. I love this web site so much, when you ask a question you will be sure to get a correct answer. I would like to wish everyone good luck and quick success [in having a baby]. – Om, 11 January 2007

In Thailand there are no support and advocacy groups formed by people around their status as infertile. This is despite the fact that Thailand has a dynamic civil society and support groups flourish for other medical conditions, such as HIV. For example, currently over nine hundred groups for people living with HIV exist with more than twenty thousand members (Lyttleton, Beesey and Sitthikriengkrai 2007). Activism by people living with HIV in Thailand on issues such as access to retroviral medicine is world famous (Ford et al. 2004, 2009).[1] Yet in Thailand there are no equivalents to the US organization RESOLVE,[2] a voluntary self-help, support and consumer advocacy group for people with infertility (Becker 2000). In the United States RESOLVE sponsors support groups, runs newsletters, has clinical advisory groups, informational meetings, telephone hotlines, evaluates and monitors physicians' performance, lobbies for legislation and disseminates information about infertility and reproductive technologies. In her ethnography of IVF in the United

States, Becker (2000) describes it as a predominantly white, middle class organization providing information for those who can afford private treatment or private adoption services. Informants in her study described the organization as a major source of support and empowerment during their treatment, expanding their knowledge of the issues and options, encouraging them to question their physicians and battle their insurance companies.

This US middle class pattern of seeking help for a health-related problem through networking and joining support groups does not seem to be replicated within Thailand's middle class. When I asked couples about their sources of information and support, they stated that their most important source of information (and for some their sole source of information) was their doctor. For example, Ploy stated: 'I did not do any research on IVF. I only rely on the doctor.' The majority of patients cited as their sources of information and advice: occasional mainstream media reports, mother and child magazines, rare TV documentaries and word of mouth from friends and family who had undergone treatment.

But for some informants, the Internet was an important source of information. For example, Laiat noted that she preferred the Internet to books for information: 'On the Internet, I have a chance to search from so many sources. There are forums with these kinds of questions and I can even learn from there.' Mon likewise frequented web boards 'where people within these problems can chat'. They typify the emergence of a new medical consumer in Thailand, one who self-educates about medical matters using information technology.

In this chapter I introduce the Thai-language online sites and chat rooms in which people seeking advice, support and information regarding infertility socialize. I systematically downloaded chat room conversations from several Thai language infertility websites from January 2007 to April 2008 and it is this data that I primarily present here. In doing so, I did not directly participate in these sites, choosing instead to observe the public texts and narratives posted to these sites, consistent with my aim of discerning the social construction and discourse framing infertility. At no point did I intrude into private 'closed' forum sites or pose as a woman seeking infertility advice (see discussion in Garcia et al. 2009).

I suggest that new forms of community are forming in cyberspace for Thai health consumers. This chapter considers the ramifications of these new forms of community and how Internet users socialize, discuss their bodies and treatments, their relationships with doctors, gender relations, and ideologies around reproduction and IVF technologies. I argue that the Internet has provided new opportunities for identifying with others who share similar biological conditions, what social scientists call 'biosociality' (Rabinow 1996). These new information technologies are contributing to reshaping how patients organize themselves into groups, construct their identities and pursue treatment.

Although there is now a substantial body of work covering many aspects of online communication, the majority of this remains centred on Internet communication in English (McLelland 2007). This Western-centric focus ignores the increasing importance of digital communication technologies in countries such as Thailand which is following the lead from sophisticated online cultures of South Korea and Japan. But access to the Internet remains the privilege of wealthy Thais who can afford computers and mobile devices. Manuel Castells (2000) has described the maldistribution in Internet access and the reinforcement of social inequalities they entail. We can be certain that most of the users of the sites I describe below are wealthy middle to upper-middle class Thais, in urban areas who can afford and have the infrastructure enabling their participation. The forms of socializing described here are simply not available to poorer rural people with fertility issues. Their ability to enter into such collectivities is limited.

Socializing in the Clinic

As many informants describe in previous chapters, undergoing IVF in Thailand can be an isolating experience. Very little socializing and information exchange takes place in clinics; patients tend to wait silently watching the ubiquitous televisions, avoiding eye contact and rarely interacting with other people. In some clinics the spatial arrangements of chairs reinforce this separation, with chairs arranged in rows rather than groupings that might encourage interaction. None of the clinics involved in this study had patient support groups to nurture the development of support or advocacy among patients.

As noted in chapter 2, partly this expresses both the secrecy and stigma still associated with infertility in Thailand and the fact that many couples wish to keep their treatment private. Likewise, the scheduling of appointments and procedures make it unlikely for patients to see each other regularly. As Pui noted: 'Most of the time, I don't meet them [patients] much. We're never here [at the clinic] at the same time. Sometimes when I am waiting for a long time we chat. But most of the time I never get to meet. I meet them once and don't meet them again.' Similarly, Pook stated, 'No, I haven't spoken to them [other patients]. Sometimes I meet the same people when I come here [to the clinic]. Sometimes I talked but never see the same person I talked to again. People who sit here don't talk. Normally you'd think they would talk, but they don't. They mind their own business.' Even those who indicated in our interviews that they would have liked to have more contact with other patients did not feel that they could initiate such contact within the clinics. People fear intrusion into their private life, as Mai said: 'I don't like others to be involved with my personal life unless they are my friends.' She also described a reluctance to give advice: 'I don't want to influence them and I feel responsible for it if the treatment is not successful for them.'

Among my informants, only an exceptional few such as Lek had exchanged phone numbers and formed relationships with other patients: 'There is not many in the group. But we don't always see each other each time. We have appointments on different days we mostly call each other. But not often. Because sometimes I don't know if they are free to pick up my call.'

Bharadwaj (2008: 107) describes Indian women in IVF clinics as so 'constrained by the overweening pronatalist patriarchal expectations the only sociality women are able to exercise is to cooperate with the discipline of clinical medicine and that of the wider joint familial network'. To a certain extent the same could be said of IVF clinics in Thailand. There is little encouragement or expectation of socializing among patients and so few opportunities or potential for relationships between them other than those defined through husbands and families, normative expectations or biomedical necessity (as with surrogates or ova donors). In addition, very little counselling takes place in Thai IVF clinics. Of the five clinics I visited and studied, only one had a dedicated nurse-counsellor (see chapter 5); others expected any counselling to take place during the invariably pressured time constraints of consultations with the physicians. Especially in public clinics, the enormous caseloads restricted the amount of time doctors could spend with patients and few patients reported having sufficient time or the fortitude to raise issues of concern with their doctors. Likewise, in informal interviews doctors lamented their inability to spend more time with patients. Patients are expected to submit to their doctors' advice and be satisfied with the information and encouragement they receive from their consultations.

'Love Clinic' and Other Internet Sites for the Infertile

In contrast to the silence that characterizes clinic encounters between people experiencing infertility, a number of Thai-language websites seem to be full of chatter. These sites include Love Clinic (clinicrak.com) which I concentrate upon in this chapter. Other such sites include weneedbaby.com, babyfancy.com, babyovutest.com and Try2conceive.forumup.com. However, Love Clinic appears to be one of the most popular; in March 2007 it was receiving 117,000 views per month. It describes itself as 'an independent homepage, not belonging to any TV channel or any certain book. It is set up to educate viewers'. Posting come from diverse locations across Thailand but also from Thai women in the United States, the United Kingdom, Australia, Japan and China. The webmaster is family welfare physician Dr Rungrort Trinit (นายแพทย์รุ่งโรจน์ ตรีนิติ).

The 'Love Clinic' website consists of a homepage with a series of links located on a prominent navigation bar. Each link denotes a family, sexual and reproductive health theme, such as sexual and reproductive health, couples relationships, children, contraception, STDs, women's problems, pregnancy, gay and lesbian issues. Clicking on the links takes the user to chat rooms on that particular topic. As will be described below, the topics of discussion within 'Love Clinic' include everything from very basic questions about the symptoms of pregnancy, how to time sexual intercourse to fall pregnant, how to conceive a baby of the appropriate sex, very technical discussions of infertility, IVF procedures and hormone regimes, frank and critical comparisons between different doctors, as well as the best sacred

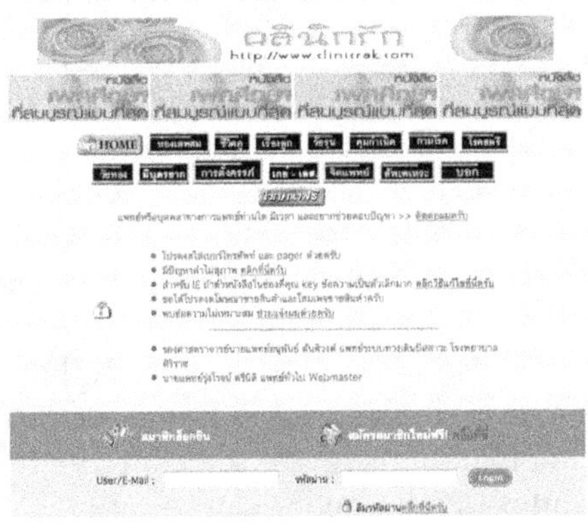

FIGURE 7.1. Web screen leading to infertility chat room in 'Love Clinic' (*clinicrak*) website.

sites for merit making and prayers, fertility diets and Chinese herbal medicines. Woven within these are stories of relationships, stigma and moral support.

Who uses these sites? Within the chat room, it appears as though the majority of participants are women, even if it is difficult to verify the gender of site users. While it is quite common to use incognitos to sign in, users often use nicknames while chatting and some email addresses are recognizable. The nicknames are usually gender identifiable and there seems to be little evidence on this site of the gender swapping (Bruckman 1996) that commonly occurs in US chatrooms and multiplayer social sites. Assuming that the web names do reflect their gender, very few 'men' make postings and those that do rarely receive any response from other participants. On the site 'Try2conceive', it was possible to print out summary statistics of the users in terms of how many visits they had made. This reveals that a small number of people participate heavily in the online discussions in a given month while the vast majority of other responders make only one response – other visitors read and make no comments. This all would appear to support an interpretation that while a vocal few actively use the internet sites as a source of biosocial interaction, the vast majority of people registered as visiting the site are passive readers only.

Remaking Nature: Cyber Biotech

These chat rooms are a rich source of information for people seeking to educate themselves about infertility or undergoing IVF and other assisted reproductive technologies. As seen in chapter 4, couples undergoing infertility treatment become highly technically conversant with the medical interventions and drug regimens and this is reflected on these sites. Discussions are dominated by technical descriptions of reproductive processes and treatments and provide insight into the ways in which the biological body becomes fragmented and divorced from the self through the technologies. Such intensified scientific and medical knowledge of their bodies is a common characteristic of 'biosocial' groups (Rose and Novas 2005). The complex descriptions of ovulation cycles, endometrial linings, ovum extractions and implantations reveal the expertise that experienced patients obtain and pass onto neophytes.

The personal stories on the site describe a litany of treatments to technological limits, as women and their doctors attempt to discipline disobedient bodies, to transform bodily functions and overcome the limitations of biology. Much discussion on this site involves the intricacies of ovarian stimulation regimes; which hormones, what timing, what to do if you've missed a dose of maturation hormone. For example, in one case 'Ono' states with technical prowess: 'Today I went to have my eggs ultrasound and I have got 38 eggs from the two sides after I injected the egg hormone Puregon 200 units for ten days. Today I injected to have the eggs mature and in another two days I have the appointment to have them collected, I'm so excited!' (15 March 2007). This is followed by a series of responses expressing their amazement, happiness, envy and hope that they will implant well: 'you will be able to do IVF so many times!' one person enthuses. Another woman in this exchange who wanted to learn more about how Ono did it left her phone number to get in touch (or was it to purchase ova from her?). Ono responds with detailed instructions as her age and medical history and the entire hormone regime she has been on.

Such stories educate patients and patients-to-be and encourage them to become active participants in their treatment. Experienced patients share their hints for timing injections, avoiding public holidays when ova extraction is due, how to save money on medicines and lore about what to do following implantation. They socialize women undergoing IVF to become savvy consumers rather than passive recipients of treatment. Through these sites, patients become aware of the full range of possibilities treatment may involve and read accounts of women who finally fall pregnant after numerous cycles of IVF.

'Can I Call You Sister?' Cyberspace Biosociality

Howard Rheingold (1993: 5) defines virtual communities as 'social aggregations that emerge from the Net when enough people carry on … public discussions long enough, with sufficient human feeling, to form webs of personal relationships in cyberspace'. 'Love Clinic' chat room members do appear to form long-term relationships with one another. It is evident that many members have been involved long term across many IVF cycles over a number of years. This community takes various forms. Members come to use closer fictive kin terms with one another, find out their ages[3] and medical histories. Throughout the chat room people gradually start to find out more about others – starting with comparing which province they are living in and what work they do, to requests to send their email addresses and phone numbers on other sites such as msn.com so that they can meet up in person or have a more intimate conversation through email. Users also offer to share leftover medicines. For example, 'Yaya' offers on 11 March 2007 to give to someone else a vial of Estrofem and Clomifene Citrate BP 50mg that she has not used. Much of the cost of IVF in Thailand is because these drugs are all imported and very expensive, so such offers represent generous gifts.

Virtual relationships also transform into real-life socializing. A group of readers decided to meet up regularly at various central well-known and accessible meeting points in Bangkok, such as the Victory monument, Central Ladprao, Central Pinklao, Future Park Rangsit, and the Night Bazaar – Lumpini Park. Thus the virtual community has spawned a real-life social support group. At another point a group from this site decided to get together in the tradition of a communal Buddhist merit-making trip, *tord pha pa,* by visiting an orphanage together and donating goods and money for its support in the anticipation that by increasing their merit in this way they would themselves become mothers. As noted in chapter 3, among patients undergoing IVF treatment, the relationship to orphanages is more for making merit directed at children to improve karma than for serious consideration of adoption as an option.

Women posting to this site share intimate details of their treatments but also their hopes, joys at successful pregnancies and sad losses. Some women state their needs simply, 'I have done five cycles now [IVF, ICSI, ZIFT] without success. I need some moral support and encouragement.' Others share their sense of devastation at failed cycles or miscarriages. The exchanges usually involve a woman posting her story and then being reassured by others in a series of supportive posts. For example, Nuu Masi wrote after another failure to fall pregnant after trying for five months of her devastation that they will have to try assisted technologies and her husband's sadness at their infertility: 'I pity my husband a lot, he does not want to do anything at all. He has never before cried, but now it's like he will not stop. I have never before experienced sadness like this before' (12 January 2007). Within fourteen minutes, her post is answered by Khun Mo who tells her: 'Be confident and patient, your doctor said it might take six months ... try to forget it and find something else to do so you don't get too stressed. The day will arrive when you will have another opportunity. Keep fighting!'

In this way the sites exert peer pressure upon participants to remain in treatment and pursue all options. They encourage those undergoing IVF to continue their treatment until all technical possibilities are exhausted and never to lose hope. In this way these sites may be seen as promoting biomedical resolution to childlessness. People posting to sites in their later stages of treatment are encouraged to pursue more and more complex interventions, such as egg donation and surrogacy. What are missing in the online accounts are women speaking of their decisions to end treatment and pursue a life without children. Such suggestions are met with rallying cries to persist. Presumably women who have decided to end their treatment simply no longer post comments nor visit the site.

However, unlike other forms of biosocial groupings around biological or disease conditions, infertility is caused by multiple factors and has various trajectories. The identity as 'infertile' is thus an unstable one; some identify it as a transitory condition for others who may have conceived a child in the past, and permanent for others. Hence, as in the exchanges above, people using this site range from those with long-term infertility problems who have been through numerous high-tech cycles to others who have failed to fall pregnant naturally and are seeking information as to whether they have a problem. The common thread linking users of these sites is the various treatment regimens and interventions rather than common underlying conditions. In the case of the infertile, as one person comments on the site, 'once people get pregnant, they move on to chat with other moms, the one who is still not pregnant is feeling left out' even while they continue to aspire to be one of those mums.

The difficult negotiations around how to handle women's descriptions of their successful pregnancies was epitomized in the discussion as to whether reading about their success itself was harmful to other women:

> Previously I visited this webboard every day and after reading what people posted to this webboard I felt stressed. So I decided to stop coming to this webboard for about two months and looked after myself. I'm not saying that this webboard is useless but it can make you feel stressed ... my husband had commented that 'the more you know and read the more stressed you are.

'WT' commented that although she had thought she would no longer visit the site, 'I am addicted!!' Yet complaints about the site are relatively rare; most people posting comments seem to find the opportunity to discuss their treatment with others helpful. For example, Pooky responded to 'WT' above that she is happy to have friends she can talk to (on the web board) as she feels the people around her are sick of hearing her.

Questioning Medical Authority

One cannot read these sites without noticing the large volume of technical talk they involve. These sites are forums for education about the pros and cons of various technologies and medications associated with infertility. Users talk of the benefits of learning from each other about the drugs and regimes of IVF so they can know what to ask their doctors and which techniques, tests and protocols they should try. As noted above, such talk positions the patient as an educated consumer, able to negotiate with and direct their physicians in their treatment. Such a position is novel in Thailand, where, as described in chapter 4, the doctor-patient relationship is overwhelmingly a patron-client relationship, with unquestioned submission to the superior status and power of the doctor. Such information thus entails more than simply education; it constitutes a political process, the empowerment of health consumers to make medical treatments more responsive to patients.

However, although the narratives of these women do indeed describe a submission to the regimes and disciplines of their clinicians, there is also evidence of resistance both to doctors' patriarchal treatment of them and to their authority. The website is a space removed from the power relationships of the clinic. Hence whole discussions centre around complaining about doctors' patronizing attitudes, lack of communication and care, expense, dismissive comments and rushed consultations. For example, one person roundly criticized a particular clinic: ' X was very sarcastic and talked down to me … if it fails again this time, we will go somewhere else … my husband never gets angry with anyone but he did not want to deal with the staff, I have to go to make the payments myself.' Another noted of one clinic: 'It's well known among patients about the "scary fat nurse" at the counter.' Doctors are freely and torridly criticized by name on the site in ways that would never happen in a face-to-face encounter. This is clearly illustrated in discussions about changing doctors. Doctors are bluntly criticized for being too busy, 'not quite thorough', not giving their contact number for emergencies, making patients 'feel intimidated to ask any questions' and the 'changing faces' they encounter in their treatment: 'His students were the ones who actually did IUI for me.… Dr X didn't do it himself.' They discuss their fear of changing doctors in case their files do not get exchanged and swap recommendations about doctors and clinics.

The website's role as a space without doctors' power was highlighted in an exchange that occurred when one person asked why there were no responses from medical doctors on the site: 'It is just all people talking with each other'. This was met with a barrage of defensive responses: 'Each website has its own purposes, why don't you try another website?'; 'This room is for people to chat and share their experiences, why don't you go see a doctor then?'; and 'I have been to so many websites, this is the best website for me and I cannot find anything like this in other websites. You can try asking questions on other website that have doctors available and see if you will get any answer. I did not get mine after waiting for the response for days.'

'Modern' Reproduction with a Traditional Twist

Part of this questioning of biomedical authority also involves the circulation of a range of other means of enhancing fertility. In chapter 3 I described the pilgrimages undertaken by Thai patients to various sacred sites to beg for babies. Such hybrid and syncretic treatment seeking is also evident in the online exchanges and reflects the multiple understandings of the body, including local humoral, religious-moral and bioscientific models, that people bring to these sites (Bharadwaj 2008: 100). While there are discussions of hormone regimes, and high-tech interventions, there are also detailed instructions of ritual procedures for asking for children from various shrines and sacred sites and invitations to meet up for joint offerings on auspicious days: 'If someone has asked for a baby from *Saan Jao Phor Seua* and succeeded, please let me know. I would like to do the same but am not quite sure how to do it.' There are transnational exchanges, with expatriate women describing auspicious sites in Japan, Hong Kong and China that may be visited.

Advice on complimentary and alternate medical treatments abound. The benefits of undertaking acupuncture at the correct time in the cycle before IUI or embryo transfer, 'to improve blood circulation', is discussed along with recommended practitioners. Likewise, Chinese herbal medicine is promoted; 'after taking fifty bags of herbal medicine I was pregnant', albeit with a warning to see a Chinese physician first before taking herbs and buying it from a trustworthy shop to ensure it does not contain steroids.

Serious discussions of astrology and fertility occur on this site, reflecting the high regard for astrology in Thai society. One woman wrote, for example, how her husband has advised her to check her horoscope before they undergo ICSI to see when she is likely to fall pregnant so that they don't waste their money on treatment. Others share stories of women who fell pregnant despite astrologers' predictions to the contrary, while another relates how 'the fortune teller told me I won't fall pregnant no matter how hard I try. It's my destiny.'

Along with astrology, dreams are often interpreted as significant portents of the future in Thailand. They reflect the religious and cultural context of treatment as well as the hopes and aspirations of infertile couples. For example:

> The other day I drove past a temple with a big Buddha image, I made a wish that 'Please I don't want to have my period this month, and please I would like to be pregnant. If my wishes are granted, I will give nine jasmine wreaths'. That night I dreamed that my husband carried a child to our car. This morning I dreamed that my husband gave me a ring with pink gemstones.... Perhaps I think about this too much.

Her account reflects her Buddhist religion and practice of promising items in return for a pregnancy described in chapter 3 (in this case the auspicious number of nine wreaths made of jasmine flowers). It also includes a more Western image of a ring with pink gemstones, an image combining Western associations of pink with girls but perhaps also the Thai association of pink with good health and perhaps the triple gems of Buddhism (the Buddha, the Dharma and the Sangha or Buddhist clergy).

Similar to the practices described in chapter 3, women posting to this site also describe how they combine multiple modalities of treatment while undergoing IVF. For example, on 1 April 2008 'Amy' described how she had tried IVF for over ten cycles, declaring, 'I went for IVF because of the expectations of my parents [to have a grandchild].' Her account detailed her attempts to make merit at various shrines while undergoing IVF treatment, including making promises to bargain at Chinese shrines, taking Chinese medicines and practicing meditation and the Dharma. She has moved from clinic to clinic and now on her most recent cycle she is pregnant – but 'not expecting much' as 'we don't dare to hope too far ahead'. The website is an opportunity for her to confidentially chat to others who have the same experience and she hopes she in turn can help her friends.

Her story is responded to by 'Baby-doll', who is also a long-term patient seeking a surrogate, and later in the conversation 'Noopu' asks 'Amy' to describe how she got pregnant on her latest attempt. 'Amy' responds that it was because of taking up regular exercise, attending a temple to practice the Dharma and meditating which made her feel calmer. She believes she might have done some bad things in her past life and that this poor karma may be why a baby doesn't want to stay with her. She also resorted to feng shui at a relative's suggestion and provides other tips such as not washing her hair herself, not using ice in her drinks or consuming soft drinks,[4] staying in bed following insertion of the embryo to assist implantation and avoiding going up and down stairs following embryo insertion until the pregnancy is well advanced. Finally, she suggests somewhat contradictory advice: 'stop thinking about it and you will get pregnant'.

Gender in the Virtual Community

There is a dominantly feminine edge to these sites. The imagery is ultrafeminine. 'Try2conceive' members decorate their postings with cute Japanese-style cartoons, pictures of babies (either their own or generic ones), pets and occasionally photographs of themselves. The threat that infertility poses for Thai women's feminine identity seems to require a strenuous reassertion of that same femininity throughout these sites.

Their identities in cyberspace are in dialogue with dominant representations of Thai women and motherhood. At times this dialogue becomes specific, such as when users engage in discussions around the stigma and discrimination they feel as women with fertility problems and the reactions of their partners. In his discussion of biosocial technologies, Rabinow (1996) notes how older cultural social categories may be reinforced by these biosocial technologies as novel modes of identification. Hence in these sites, normative notions of Thai femininity as equated with motherhood and nurturance powerfully intersect with the quest for an IVF baby. This has also been observed for IVF clinics in India where long-standing pressures for women to conceive are a defining feature of the way women's bodies within the clinic are presented (Bharadwaj 2008).

Likewise, many of the users on these sites invoke and reinforce Thai gender stereotypes in their depictions of motherhood. For example, discussions often reinforce pronatalist discourses of gender roles and the importance of motherhood for defining womanhood. Women encourage each other to submit to the hardships of treatment and 'continue to fight for a child'. They are urged to 'give up everything', in order to 'just have someone call you Mum'. Occasionally, users question this. Commenting on the suggestion that women undergoing IVF should give up work, 'Amy' notes (1 April), 'not working doesn't mean you will get pregnant'.

However, the sites do reveal the gendered tensions surrounding infertility in Thai society. For example 'Nop' below explains that even though they are using ICSI because of her partner's infertility, he has asked her to promise not to reveal his infertility to anyone. She writes: 'It's so hard being a woman ... when I did not have a boyfriend, people asked me when I would have one, when I have one, people asked me when I was getting married and when I am married, people still ask when I will be pregnant! (Do you know how stressful this is??????).'

Many women speak of their need to produce a son and heir for their husbands, pressure from grandparents and inheritance concerns as the reasons for pursuing assisted reproductive technologies. These technologies are consumed not only for individual fulfilment but also for gendered familial obligations. One woman wrote of how her treatment is due to her husband's infertility, yet she is not allowed to reveal this to anyone and as a result is blamed by her in-laws for the lack of children – they are encouraging him to divorce her. Another woman feels she has failed her husband: 'I feel very sorry for my husband because I know that he really wants to have a child and I cannot provide that for him. If I really cannot give him a baby, I would want him to be with somebody else.' Another woman writes: 'I feel so sorry for my husband.... I never cried but up to this point, I don't know if I can take it anymore. I have never felt so weak before.' The stresses of treatment also take their toll on relationships. As one woman writes: 'Only people in here [this chat room] understand me. I used to get excited with my husband [about implantation]. Now, he told me to let him know whenever it's really for sure [pregnant].... I don't know who I should talk to now.'

The strains to relationships are evident in accounts from women of men threatening divorce or to take 'minor' wives to produce an heir. In response to a question from a male writer on whether a man with one testicle can still have a baby, another discussant drily observed: 'My husband has one ball but was able to make 2 women pregnant at the same time.' Such frank, even crude intimate discussions of relationships to strangers are unusual in Thai society where polite norms of social interaction and face saving according to status and relationship are carefully observed. In the digital space, however, there exists an anonymous freedom allowing women to verbalize issues that would be difficult to do in other settings.

Biosociality

In his study of the Human Genome project, Rabinow suggested that the 'infiltration of techno-science, capitalism and culture into 'nature" (1996: 103) will lead to the 'likely formation of new group and individual identities and practices' (1996: 102). In its simplest form, biosociality refers to collective identities emerging from categories in biomedicine and science (Rapp 1999: 302). The concept of biosociality has led to a range of projects concerned with how biotechnologies are reshaping how humans understand themselves, create their identities, their relations to others, their experiences and expectations of health, illness and embodiment and their interrelations with capitalism (Ong and Chen 2010; Ong and Collier 2005).

In sites such as 'Love Clinic' we see an example of the interface between two new technologies, medically assisted reproduction and the Internet and resultant forms of collective identity making. Cyberspace allows forms of association between people with fertility difficulties unavailable in other spaces. The Internet offers a form of virtual community for people for whom no other forums for sociality exists. As I have described above, on these Internet sites we see evidence of the development of forms of identity in which infertility and various technological interventions becomes the dominant narrative.

Nikolas Rose and Carlos Novas (2005) suggest that biosocial groups should be defined as those that entail particular relationships with the state, 'biological citizenship'. Deborah Heath, Rayna Rapp and Karen-Sue Taussig (2004) note such citizenship is manifested in struggles over individual identities, collectivization, access to knowledge, demands for recognition and claims to expertise and a new ethics and politics of embodied experience. They have subdivided various forms of biocitizenship such as 'informational biocitizenship', in which groups lobby for better treatment, patient rights or funding for research, or 'digital biocitizenship' in which communities are linked electronically. In short, organizations such as RESOLVE are paradigmatic examples asserting biological citizenship as they not only socialize, but share information, lobby government and promote patient empowerment.

For Veena Das in India the concept of biosociality as the 'forming of associational communities to influence state policy and science' has little relevance among impoverished Delhi subalterns as it presumes 'the individual as the subject of a liberal political regime' (2001: 2). In a similar vein, in her work on IVF clinics in Ecuador, Elizabeth Roberts (2008) questions the assumptions behind the notion of the 'social' in biosociality. She argues that the lack of a civil society in Ecuador and the nature of its history and politics results in an absence of activist patients groups advocating for themselves as liberal subjects in relation to the state.

To what extent does the virtual community of *Love Clinic* and associated sites entail particular relationships with the Thai state? Bharadwaj (2008: 100) suggests that the concept of biosociality 'is limited in the global context ... and perhaps as a concept it was never intended to travel very far in the first place'. As noted by Das and Roberts, it may be that the forms of biosocial groupings RESOLVE represents are particular to Western cultures and that such forms of sociality are simply not applicable cross-culturally, based as they are on certain forms of liberal democracy and a degree of economic and social capital. Yet Thailand has a dynamic civil society with numerous groups asserting their needs and rights, including groups based around medical issues such as HIV (Ford et al. 2009). The space and model for activism is thus well established in Thai society.

But such activism is usually associated with underprivileged and discriminated groups in Thailand who must fight for recognition of their rights and livelihoods. We might question why these particular virtual communities lack the transformative power evident for other biosocial groupings in Thai society. Unlike the subaltern communities described by Das, we know users with internet access are wealthy and well educated people who might be expected to have the means to organize more advocacy. However, in Thailand it is rare for the middle to upper middle classes to be involved in such groups as they rarely find their interests in opposition to those of the Thai state. Class then may be one reason why the privileged seekers of infertility treatment do not lobby more actively and transform their nascent biosociality into more overt political forms. The only political statement made on the online sites during the monitoring period referred to the costs of treatment and the fact that Thailand does not provide any schemes to assist with the cost of infertility treatment which is considered 'elective'. This was contrasted by one woman posting to 'Love Clinic' with the massive state support of family planning; she wants the Thai government to consider infertility as a problem: 'They only concentrate on a "birth control".' Yet there is little evidence of activism or advocacy by patients in either clinics or on infertility Internet sites.

Until recently, another condition that discouraged the formation of further advocacy or activism was the lack of regulations in Thailand to IVF treatment. Access to treatment in Thailand remains a privilege of the wealthy and the Thai state does not offer state financial support for high-tech assisted reproductive technologies but also did not restrict their use until 2015. In short, infertility patients at the time of writing had few state regulations to advocate for or against. The only restrictions on treatment involved their capacity to pay. It is possible that the advent of state regulations will promote advocacy. For example, restrictions in the forthcoming legislation restricting commercial ova donation or commercial surrogacy (discussed in chapter 9) will limit the choices people have for treatment.

A further barrier to the growth of advocacy is the stigma of infertility particularly as it involves a couple. Chatting on a web board is one thing, publically announcing infertility or openly attending a support group meeting is another entirely. Some celebrities have 'come out' as seeking or using assisted reproductive technologies, providing opportunities for public education and discussion of the technologies, but for the most part such treatment remains discrete and private. Online communities facilitate anonymous interactions and 'informational biosociality', but in the absence of a catalyst may never transform into a more advocacy-based organization.

Finally, other factors may be working against the growth of activism. Throughout the IVF industry and replicated on these sites is the discourse that stresses faith in technology and a sense that infertility is a temporary condition of individuals that will eventually be fixed by bioscience. Perhaps this mitigates against complete adoption of infertility as an identity term. Just as one's identity as infertile may be transitory, online communities are transitory. Further, these sites reinforce the gendered identities of women as mothers or mothers-to-be. They generally encourage women to fulfil their roles as mothers, not through fighting for patient rights or state support, but through diligent submission to the discipline of IVF treatment and their doctor's advice.

The kinds of biosociality found in the United States, Europe and Australia, in groups such as RESOLVE, are not merely products of access to certain communication technologies, but are linked to particular conceptions of citizenship and personhood. They connect to histories of political activism, vociferous identity politics and an ideology of active self-fulfilment (Rose 2007: 147). Infertile biosociality in Thailand takes a muted form compared to that in the United States; within cyberspace it is oriented towards information sharing, consumer education and moral support, it promotes hope rather than contesting medical expertise or seeking redress from the state. But we should not dismiss the importance of these sites as a means for Thais to develop new forms of association. In their own small ways, the women and men visiting these Thai-language internet sites are developing what Rose (2007: 146) terms 'a new informed ethics of the self – a set of techniques for managing everyday life in relation to a condition, and in relation to expert knowledge'. It does represent a new relationship with biomedicine for Thai patients; no longer the uninformed passive patient, users of these sites are educating themselves about the technologies, learning to assert their wishes and negotiate with their doctors. They are reflecting upon gender relations and being exposed to the stories, concerns and support of their fellow patients in ways which the clinics themselves do not encourage or facilitate.

Notes

1. In 1999 the Thai Government Pharmaceutical Organization (GPO) sought a compulsory licence from the Thai Department of Intellectual Property in order to produce a generic version of Didanosine for the treatment 700,000 Thai HIV/AIDS patients. This request was supported by local NGOs, the Thai Network for People living with HIV/AIDS (TNP+) and Médecins Sans Frontières (MSF). Under threats of trade sanctions against Thailand from the US government, the Thai Commerce Ministry refused the licence. In May 2001 the Thai AIDS Access Foundation, together with two people living with HIV/AIDS, filed the lawsuit against the Bristol-Myers Squibb (BMS) patent. Their victory in obtaining this ruling demonstrates that the right to health and the right to life can be protected by challenging patents and not yielding to threats from industrialized countries. In practical terms the ruling means that the GPO should now be able to produce a generic formula of Didanosine at considerable cost savings to HIV/AIDS patients.
2. Established in 1974, RESOLVE is The National Infertility Association, a nationwide nonprofit organization to promote reproductive health and to ensure equal access to all family building options for men and women experiencing infertility or other reproductive disorders.

3. Asking one's age is a vital step in Thai society where appropriate terms of address rely upon understanding the social hierarchy between elder and younger people.
4. These proscriptions against ice drinks refer to humoral models of the body in which fertile women need to maintain a 'heated state' which could be shocked by imbibing overly cold substances.

Chapter 8

'Technology That Gives Men Hope'

Little has been written about the experiences of men engaging with reproductive technologies; for the most part ethnographic and qualitative studies of reproduction have focussed on women and been undertaken by female researchers. The overall paucity of studies concentrating upon men's experiences may be due to the reported tendency of men to underreport in studies on reproductive matters (Inhorn 1996). Within the literature on assisted reproduction there has been a tendency to depict men's involvement in IVF as relatively minor, ignoring both the lived experience and subjectivity of infertile men (Inhorn 2004b). Since the introduction of new invasive technologies for the treatment of male factor infertility, such a view of men's involvement is inadequate (Inhorn 2007b: 39). More studies focussing on men's embodiment of these technologies are required. The social science literature of reproduction is filled with studies of women's reproductive lives, through the eyes of women, not from men themselves (van Balen and Inhorn 2002).

Such neglect of men's experiences of infertility belies the fact that male factors such as low sperm count, poor sperm motility, defective sperm morphology and an absence of sperm in the ejaculate affect more than half of all cases of infertility. Almost 30 per cent of cases of infertility are caused solely by male factors (Isidori, Latini and Romanelli 2005). Results of the causes of infertility of 1,072 couples treated at the infertility clinic of Thammasat Hospital in Bangkok between 1999 and 2004 reveal that 19.4 per cent of couples were treated for male factor infertility only, while a further 55.6 per cent of couples had both male and female factors, and 17.5 per cent had female factors only (Chaimchanya and Su-angkawatin 2008).

Like their female counterparts, infertile men suffer from social stigma (Becker 2000). A prolonged absence of children is discrediting to a couple. As discussed in chapter 2, many men find the experience of infertility and its treatment as profoundly threatening to their sense of masculinity. A number of studies document how infertile men attempt to reconcile their experiences with cultural expectations. Marcia Inhorn and Emily Wentzell (2011) describe the complex ways men negotiate, reject or reinvent locally hegemonic forms of manhood in response to the advent of new reproductive technologies. Men's reactions to these technologies demonstrate how men's real lives are often far different from local stereotypes.

This chapter provides further comparative material for a consideration of how men engage with reproductive technologies and the implications for their performance of masculinity. In particular it describes men's involvement in the treatment of themselves and their partners.

Thai Masculinity

Studies of gender and sexualities in Thailand note the diversity and fluidity of genders and sexualities in Thailand and the ways in which they are being contested and changed in the context of rapid social change and global engagement (Jackson and Cook 1999). Thai gender[1] is best represented as a continuum, in which masculinity, regardless of sexual orientation, is celebrated as active rather than passive, strong and powerful.[2] Age, status and ethnicity all interact to reinforce gendered identities to produce multiple ways in which masculinity is demonstrated and performed. Multiple stereotypes of Thai male ideals are common in the press and social media, linked by a common depiction of masculine power and authority: from hard-working, physically strong, independent, skilled and resilient peasant farmers and tough, disciplined *muay Thai* fighters through to middle class ideals of a suave, well-groomed, authoritative businessman to the respected disciplined benevolent power of monks.

Demonstrations of masculine power include displays of wealth involving consumption of food, drink and women, and influence over dependents such as employees. As Graham Fordham (2004) has noted, for many Thai men displays of masculine identity involve feasting, drinking and occasional forays to brothels. He suggests that for Thai men such occasions provide opportunities for the display of their merit, status and prowess, competitive displays of drinking capacity and maintaining bodily control. A sexual double standard pervades Thai relationships, with the perception that men have a natural and strong sexual desire and need for varied and frequent intercourse. Thai women are sometimes willing to tolerate or ignore men's extramarital sexual encounters, particularly if it does not involve ongoing emotional or material obligations (Knodel et al. 1999; Packard-Winkler 1996).

The depicted normative ideal of male-female relations is of a dominant male to a highly submissive female (Muecke 1992). Although women are highly visible in public life and employment, men generally enjoy social privilege and superior opportunities to women. Men are officially defined as heads of a household and generally considered to take the leadership in public affairs while women dominate the domestic (and reproductive) realm. Thai notions of appropriate senior-junior (*phi-nong*) positioning affect gender relations. For example, a wife is expected to defer to her husband's authority in public. All the women of this study were married to older men, consistent with this cultural expectation of the seniority of the male partner.

Male Involvement in Treatment

As described in chapter 4, within the clinics I observed women were the focus of medical attention. The demands of IVF treatment meant that women had to attend the clinics regularly, while men were usually only required to visit occasionally. Most men were willing to accompany their wives to seek care, although, as in the case of Mai, women were usually the ones to seek care initially: 'It was my idea to come to this hospital. I came here myself to chat with the doctor and nurses. Then I had a chat with my husband and dragged him down here. He could not refuse.'

Some men reported very little involvement in the IVF procedures which focus upon women even in cases of male infertility. In one case involving an expatriate couple coming from overseas for treatment, the husband merely visited the clinic once to deposit a sperm sample and then returned overseas, leaving his wife to continue treatment. Most did not accompany their partners to all appointments, either due to the difficulties of getting time off work for the numerous appointments or due to the sense that their presence was unnecessary. Many of the men interviewed expressed a deep commitment to their wives and a desire to support them through the treatment. Some viewed their role as primarily financial, many taking on extra work so that their wives could undertake IVF, especially as many women gave up work to undertake treatment.

A range of clinic practices that excluded men was a further barrier to their involvement with the treatments. For example, none of the clinics I observed allowed male partners to accompany their female partners for intrauterine insemination (IUI), or the surgical retrieval of ovum, despite many women stating they would have liked to have their partners be present to hold their hands. As I observed in my earlier work on birthing in Thailand, such arbitrary exclusion of men is also common in many hospitals for women giving birth. Clinic nurses stated that women would be too embarrassed to have their partners present through such intimate procedures. The clinic Mot attended did allow men to be present during vaginal ultrasounds if they wished:

> But when I had my birth canal ultrasounded, I asked if he wanted to go in but he was not comfortable to. I called him in many times but he refused. He said that he would wait until the ultrasound of my [pregnant] tummy. He was embarrassed to see the doctor doing the procedure on me. For us, women, we want our husband to be by our side for moral support because a nurse took me into a room and put me on the table and left. The doctor came to give the injection [IUI] and left. I was just lying there alone.

One clinic explained to me that it was not possible to have partners present for the fact that a number of women were treated in close proximity and there was a risk that anyone present might inadvertently see other women in treatment. Men were assigned to the waiting room.

One way in which men involved themselves was through modifying their lifestyles. Men reported following their doctor's recommendations to reduce their smoking and drinking, watch their diets, work less and relax more to improve the quality of their sperm. Jon's discovery of his infertility caused him to consider his lifestyle and health:

> I have not quit smoking yet but smoke less now because I think of my wife. I used to smoke about two packets a day. While I was working at the site, I would light a cigarette because I had nothing else to do. I only smoke a little bit then threw it away. At home, my wife would remind me to stop. I must admit that I have decreased the amount of cigarettes from two packets a day to eight to ten cigarettes a day. Sometimes, I don't even finish the whole cigarette.... [But] It's still difficult for me to quit completely.

Like their wives, men reported eating foods understood in Thailand to improve fertility such as oysters, sesame seeds and avoiding tofu. Jon was taking vitamins B and C and bitter melon to improve his sperm. Teranit spoke of other traditional techniques to improve his fertility, claiming efficacious herbal treatments existed in Indonesia and India. Faa noted:

> Lots of people advised us to eat certain foods, eat this! Don't eat that! To help increase the sperm count and so we did ... all the time but we know after that it is a problem with the workings of the testicles [that produces the sperm], nothing to do with the food we have eaten in the last three years. We used to take vitamin E and avoid Chinese celery and eat holy basil [*horapha*] a lot and avoid soya milk. But it hasn't worked.

Collecting Sperm

For many men in the study, providing sperm samples was the only intervention in which they participated. Sperm collection through masturbation was a cause of acute embarrassment for male patients and some women reported that their husbands were reticent to discuss the procedure with them at all. The stress of producing a sperm sample is heightened by the pressure to produce it at a prescribed time. Similar issues are reported for Israeli and Canadian men in fertility treatment (Carmeli and Birenbaum-Carmeli 1994). In Egypt and Lebanon, Inhorn (2007b) reports on the shame associated with masturbation for Muslim men. Religious-based injunctions against masturbation produce guilt for many Muslim men asked to produce semen samples. Masturbation is regarded as distasteful and sinful and semen as defiling. The need to obtain semen samples through masturbation in the clinics she studied was further hindered by local prohibitions on pornography and the lack of private intimate spaces for semen collection (Inhorn 2007b). Although in the Thai context there seems to be less anxiety over masturbation, nevertheless Manit felt the need to explain how he differentiated between masturbation associated with sexual pleasure and that undertaken for sperm collection. Using Buddhist philosophy, he explained that the difference lay in the consciousness within which the act was undertaken: 'I keep asking sacred things. I didn't collect sperm out of lust. Before I collected sperm I prayed that what I am about to collect be a good act out of which good things may come. I asked that good things may come out of what I am about to collect. So I had consciousness in what I was doing.'

Each clinic in the study had a room allocated for sperm collection, usually equipped with adult magazines and pornographic videos (although one public clinic reported that the pornography was repeatedly stolen). However, both Ploy and Mon reported that at two provincial hospitals they had attended for treatment their husbands had been forced to collect sperm in the public toilet as there was no collection room. Tuk's husband also used the public toilet, as the collection room was occupied. Even at clinics with private rooms, some were not liked by men as they were publically visible within the clinics so everyone in the clinic knew where you were going and what you were about to do. Bunmi explained:

> It is characteristic of Thai men that they are ashamed [about this]. If it is possible the hospital staff should call to see them inside, not hand me a container in front of a lot of people. Sometimes it has a psychological effect. When I collect sperm I shouldn't be stressed and embarrassed but I felt all of this. It should be more discreet. The room is not really supportive for me to create the right mood to collect sperm. And this creates difficulties. There is nothing to help me. Then I have to walk past a lot of people with the container. We all know we are here for the treatment but naturally it is embarrassing. If we are called to go inside we should just enter they don't have to give me anything so others can see.... It makes people who come from treatment feel embarrassed.

Ton did not worry about being seen by other patients, however he suffered embarrassment when he handed over his sample: 'I felt an inferiority complex that I had such a small amount of sperm especially when I had to hand it to a nurse. For other [men], they might think of it as a male problem and it's such a disgrace for them.'

The best arrangement men reported was in a private hospital where the collection room was on a separate floor so men were spared the parade in front of the other patients:

> I have collected sperm at a lot of hospitals now. The best was hospital C. It had the best sperm collection room. It had the most privacy. The room had two doors. Here at B if the door gets opened there is only one door but in hospital C there were two. The room itself isn't much different. It has movies, stuff like that. At hospital C they have everything. Good books, everything. But here they have only one CD. But there [at C] they have lots of different things. Their equipment is better. (Withoon)

Apart from the public visibility of the entrance to the sperm collection room, men reported difficulty with the video equipment at one clinic, accidentally spilling semen and not being sure that the switch was working that indicates to hospital staff that a sample was ready. Ton explained:

> The place is good however the [video] equipment in the collecting room did not work both times I used it. It can be a problem because the equipment helps a man to feel aroused.... The first time, the player worked but there were no CDs, so the second time, I prepared my own CDs but the player was broken. I thought it was funny but it was still a problem. I feel that they did not pay good attention to the room.

Such incidents further added to the sense of emasculation and depersonalization experienced by men in the treatment process. Some women reported that their husbands refused to participate further due to the humiliation they felt.

Men's Attitudes towards Donor Sperm

Interviews with the Thai men in this study revealed an intense reluctance to use donor sperm. Men had stronger feelings about the need for a biological tie than the women interviewed. As Becker (2000) noted, assisted reproductive technologies maintain the emphasis on biological relatedness which makes it more difficult for women and men to contemplate nonbiological parenthood. The advent of ICSI and TESE/PESA techniques in the 1990s that allow for the removal of spermatozoa directly from the testicles or epididymis and subsequent injection of a single spermatozoon directly into an ovum has reinforced the importance of paternity. These techniques create the possibility that even a severely infertile man may father a genetic offspring. ICSI has quickly spread throughout IVF clinics in Thailand since its introduction in 1999 (Choavaratana, Suppinyopong and Chaimahaphruksa 1999). As one embryologist noted, demand for donated sperm has decreased with the new technology of ICSI such that now 'patients would not use it unless they have no other choices'. 'They would prefer to use their own reproductive cells first', unless they were so financially constrained they could not afford to undertake ICSI or there was no alternative. Teranit stated: 'In the case of a woman, [in the case of ovum donation] even though it is someone else's egg but my wife is the one to carry the baby, if you ask her, "Is that OK?" Then "[Yes, it is] OK." But it must be my sperm. As far as I know if there is nothing wrong with the semen we can get the sperm from the testicles [TESE] so I stopped thinking about using donated sperms.'

Later he added: 'For myself I insist it must be my sperm. Otherwise I won't raise the child.' Only one couple in this study was using anonymous donated sperm at the time of our interview. Phet 'didn't have a problem' with using donor sperm, as she felt it 'would still be our baby. That's right. My egg, my child, right?' She explained that the doctor would choose the sperm most appropriate for their use 'from a man who has a similar skin colour, same blood group as his [her husband] and double eyelids with straight hair, et cetera. We are not allowed to be too picky. I had a concern about IQ but I am not allowed to be picky so I don't know about the IQ level.' According to one clinic's embryologist, sperm is supplied from a local service centre where all donors were screened for various transmissible diseases and all were required to have, at minimum, a bachelor's degree. The donations were then classified into blood groups, skin colours, heights and quality of sperms.

For most men, however, the idea of using donated sperm was rejected. The importance of genetic relatedness was expressed by reference to the family 'bloodline' (*say luad rao,* สายเลือดเรา). Ton said he would not contemplate using donated sperm despite his infertility: 'In my opinion, "our child" is someone who descends from us. I am talking about the same DNA so I would be able to call them "ours". If not, it's a human but not "our child". At least, I want someone who has the same blood; for example, I would prefer adopting our brothers' or sisters' child.'

Ut and Khiat had contemplated donor insemination at a previous clinic. They had decided that 'if worse came to worse', they would try insemination with Khiat's brother's sperm in order to maintain the family relatedness. 'Going with the family' was viewed as preferable to utilizing an anonymous donor. However, once they heard about the availability of ICSI at their present clinic, they abandoned that plan.

Surprisingly, for all the concern expressed by men about the importance of genetic relatedness, few were aware of or had asked about clinic procedures for ensuring that there were no mix-ups between sperm and egg samples in the laboratory. All clinics followed protocols for labelling and confirming that correct gametes were used, but they confirmed that few patients ever asked about the procedures used. This contrasts, for example, to reports from Israeli clinics where for religious reasons patients expressed grave concerns over the possible mixing up of gametes (Kahn 2000). When asked about the processes for ensuring that no mistakes were made, Manit replied that is was largely a matter of trust in the ethics of the health staff: 'In fact it is difficult to prove whether it's our sperm or another [person's]. Although they say, "yes, it is yours", but it is something you can't see because they don't let you follow them all the time. Like my sperm I gave it to the nurse, she gives it to the lab. We don't follow every single step so to say "yes" or "no" it is hard to say so.' He reasoned that if they did use other people's sperm then they would have a higher success rate: 'Like all the cases would be successful wouldn't they? Why would only some conceive, only some. It must be our sperm.... Because each successful case brings fame to the hospital, those that are not successful it is like the other edge of the sword, because unsuccessful cases will try again and the hospital makes more money. Anyway I believe they wouldn't do that.'

He had been reassured by a CD they received of the procedure: 'It's our CD and the doctor confirmed that this is all our eggs and all our sperm.'

The Experience of ICSI and TESE

The growth of ICSI speaks of the willingness of both women and men to undergo invasive interventions in order to conceive. Intracytoplasmic sperm injection (ICSI) now allows infertile men to produce biologically related children. Khiat described ICSI as 'a technology that gives men hope'. As a result of the development of ICSI, there is pressure on women to undergo the arduous experience of IVF and ICSI procedures, even when the male partner is the one with the infertility problem, rather than using the simpler, less expensive and less invasive intervention of IUI with donor sperm. In the Middle East, Inhorn has shown how the advent of ICSI has led to both increased hope for men but also increased suffering as otherwise fertile women undergo IVF cycles. She found that in some cases men requiring ICSI would divorce their older wives to seek younger wives to increase their chances of a successful ICSI cycle (Inhorn 2003a).

ICSI requires women to undergo a full cycle of IVF, including hormonal stimulation, oocyte retrieval and embryo transfer, even if they have no fertility issues. Judith Lorber (1989) suggests that in many cases, a woman's subordinate status in the marital relationships combined with pressure from physicians means that women in these circumstances may be making a 'patriarchal bargain' rather than a free choice or freely given gift. A woman may feel she has little choice other than to undergo treatment, despite the risks to her own health and fertility, if she wishes to maintain her relationship with her husband. Sacrifice and altruism is expected for motherhood. Lorber suggests fertility doctors take for granted that women will want to undertake the high-tech procedures and rarely question women's motivations.[3]

Women who were undertaking IVF for their husband's infertility stated it was because they wanted to provide a biological child for their husband, or because he was 'a good husband'. Most of the men interviewed seemed to take it for granted that their wives would undergo IVF to produce a biologically related child with them. Jon was one of the few men to comment on the arduous process his wife was undergoing to undertake ICSI because of his infertility and the emotional commitment this demonstrated: 'I think of her when she has to go through pains and surgeries. I feel sorry for her.' For many men, ICSI requires invasive interventions as well, especially when surgical removal of spermatozoa from the testes (TESE) is required. Few men were willing to go into detail about their experience with these operations, instead preferring to stoically dismiss their pain and discomfort. Lek described her husband's experience:

> The first time he had surgery to take the testicle tissue out to check in the lab to see if there are any sperms. And there were. Then we had to wait anxiously to see if they were strong and healthy. If they were not complete, not straight, we may have to waste our money for nothing. He was stressed then. The second cycle that we started he was afraid whether it will feel the same again because he felt like he had been punched. After the first time when the testicle had been cut he couldn't walk it was stiff and then we had to wait anxiously to see if there are sperms on the other side [other testicle] as well.

Khiat and his wife were pregnant following ICSI. Although they considered using his brother's sperm to conceive a baby, they were relieved that TESE/ICSI offered the opportunity for Khiat to try to father his child. He did not mind the pain of the TESE procedure, explaining that on the day of his TESE procedure he was 'scared initially but when the time came, I was surprisingly calm. I am usually easily scared but on the day, I did not feel anything. Other people worried more about me having the operation but I felt fearless. Perhaps, I could see a chance of success.' He has since told other men at work about ICSI: 'If he has the same problem, I would tell him not to lose hope altogether. I used to think that it was impossible [for me to father a child] but it was not like that. There are ways to help. I believe that every man can have a baby but they might need a little assistance from the doctor and they have to prepare for be in pain. Anyway, it will be worth the pain.'

Teranit

A case study of Teranit provides a deeper understanding of the complexities and negotiations involved for men in treatment for infertility. We interviewed Teranit while he waited for his wife to come from her consultation. He was frank in his discussion but concerned that the details would remain anonymous. After interviewing Teranit, we were able to interview his wife. Teranit is an airline pilot, age forty-one, and his wife, Nong, is thirty-nine. They were married in 1996 and although they immediately tried to start a family had not fallen pregnant after a year without using contraceptives so they went to see a doctor in a regional town. The doctor discovered that Teranit had a low sperm count and prescribed some medicine which he took for two months. They fell pregnant but tragically discovered the child was carrying a devastating genetic abnormality (anencephaly) and were forced to abort five months into their pregnancy. Teranit explained that following the tragic termination they did not try to fall pregnant again for six years:

> We weren't brave enough to have another child because the doctor said if we had another we would have the same problem. So we stopped for a long time. Really, if we hadn't stopped and fell pregnant it is possible there wouldn't be a problem but we were scared. And then during that time we felt the family wasn't complete without a baby and so we tried again in 2003.

As with other men in this research, Teranit is careful about to whom he discloses his infertility: 'If they are close friends I tell them but in this society they don't ask. I have never come across someone asking me, "Are you abnormal?" Never.' He admitted that he feels different to other male friends:

> Really, I do feel a little bit [different]. All my friends in my cohort have all got children. They tease me while we are drinking that 'I have to change the mother of the child' something like that.... They just tease me. My close friends ask when will I have [a child] ... but

> people who aren't close, when they know I have a problem they don't ask any further questions. They won't go into further details. This is a private issue.

After two unsuccessful attempts with IUI, a doctor at a military hospital advised Teranit to undertake ICSI due to his poor sperm count. They tried ICSI twice without success at another hospital. He then went abroad to work for a year and explained that during that time he had separated from his wife due to an extramarital affair: 'The last year I worked abroad for the year and after [that] I decided [to try to have a child]. My wife suggested that if we couldn't do it [have a child], she would leave and we also had another problem to do with a girlfriend ... so we have to do it to be a family and even though we need to spend money, here we are.' Undertaking another round of ICSI and having a biological child was thus described as something which was important to keep their relationship together:

> At that time I believed in horoscopes. And the fortune teller told us to try at a hospital with a foreign name. So we went to X hospital. My wife asked me to have an examination and then they found that I had a varicose vein in my testicles. And so I had surgery. After I recovered my semen improved. I just got to know the result the other day. At first there was a problem with the head of the sperm, a 'head defect.' The head was too big it couldn't get into the egg by itself. But now the head defect has decreased and is normal now. But the sperm count is still the same. It has only improved just slightly probably because I am old.

The varicocelectomy Teranit underwent refers to a painful testicular operation to remove a 'varicocele', a dilation of the scrotal veins draining the testes. Teranit attributes an improvement to his sperm morphology to his operation. Treatment of varicocele remains controversial and there is no agreement as to whether it is of any benefit (Isidori, Latini and Romanelli 2005: 315). Inhorn (2007a) notes that, despite the uncertainty, such operations continue to be commonly undergone by infertile men in the Middle East. Further research is required to find out how common such operations are in men's treatment in Thailand.

As with most couples in this study, the costs of treatment have been considerable. In their case, Teranit estimated the costs, to date, at 500,000 baht (approximately US $16,000). Patients are aware that private clinics have vested interests in their treatment and patients sometimes query why some procedures have been suggested despite their low chances of success. In his case he questioned why a previous clinic had asked him to use a frozen sperm sample despite knowing its lower chances of success: 'So I wonder why they ask me to do it. Make me waste money. Private hospitals should know that it isn't good and shouldn't use this method with us, hey? This is what I think. Maybe they just want my money.' Their current treatment is complicated due to the fact that his wife is now in her late thirties. This has complicated their treatment but Teranit also noted that it has brought less blame to him as 'she has a problem too now.... We will use donated eggs now. We have to find someone who will give us some eggs. We won't treat my wife anymore, use donated eggs. I just spoke to my wife and she has someone in mind already.'

Although both he and his wife accepted the notion of using a donated egg, as noted earlier, Teranit would never accept the use of donated sperm. When asked about his feelings about having a child he responded:

> I think it is a good thing because it helps complete a family. Because when you are aged, like me, you can say that I am successful in my career and then there will be women hitting on me. If our family is not complete and not strong enough, then it is likely that I will make such a mistake – wasting money on women, [when] I should have a child. So having treatment is a good thing. It is the right way. If I don't have a child I will have a problem [womanizing]. If I don't have a baby then I don't know who I am working for. I think it is necessary to have a complete family.

Teranit and his wife tried to care for a seven-year-old nephew for almost two years. This form of informal adoption within families is common in Thailand, but in their case it was problematic. They found his behaviour difficult and demanding. This caused strains within their marriage and in their family relationships.

> Yes, it has had a lot of effect [on our relationship]. Because my wife brought a nephew home to live. And his behaviour was unbearable. Taking the nephew we brought all his problems and all of my wife's family as well.... I was ready to divorce. Because we took him in he started demanding things of us. He wasn't our child. This problem carried on until the end. In the end I didn't want him and so he had to leave. We bought him a motorcycle and we are still paying it off. There are a lot of problems if you don't have a baby [of your own]. ... Even if he was good, his parents might still come.... If we raise him we would expect a lot from him, want him to be this, be that,

> but he isn't our child. When we had problems and quarrelled with his parents they took their son back and now they ignore us and my wife stays by herself because I work overseas, work for two months and return for two weeks. When he left he took everything with him. Abandoned us to stay by ourselves like old people. They didn't consider the time and money we spent supporting him.

Although he claimed there was no pressure on him to have a child as his parents have passed away, Teranit spoke of the pressure his wife feels, exacerbated by the difficulties it has caused on their relationship:

> My wife might have some pressure because she has experience about this [from her previous pregnancy]. Because we don't have a baby of our own we have to rely on others. We separated for a long time, for a year because of this problem, plus I had another person in my life. For me I want to have a child to make my family complete, but my wife *must* have one. Because if she doesn't have one she is not complete.... She must have her own baby. When we broke up she used to think of finding another man but now she knows she also has a problem [with her fertility]. So both sides, the man and woman both have problems so it makes it even more difficult.

Upon questioning about their previous pregnancy, Teranit admitted that he had been disappointed initially with the pregnancy upon finding out that the embryo was a girl:

> It was a girl. We got to see the gender from the first ultrasound but we didn't know there was something wrong with the skull. Then I came home and got drunk. I am sorry.... I wanted a boy. At that time the next day [I was thinking] have we made the wrong decision? And five months later we went back and then we didn't even have a girl. We went to Chula hospital for the test for the 3D ultrasound. The doctor couldn't confirm the problem so he went for the ultrasound at Chula and then sent the records to [the regional town]. Then he told us.

Teranit's case reminds us of the lived complexities of men and women's reproductive lives. A tragic reproductive loss of a first pregnancy following initial fertility treatment had caused delays to further attempts which affected the couple's fertility further. He felt guilty over his initial disappointment at having conceived a girl on their first pregnancy, only to later find out that the pregnancy required a medical termination due to devastating genetic problems. This event had affected the couple deeply. As with other couples in this study, children are seen as an essential element to bind the relationship between the couple together and as companions in old age. For Teranit, a child also represents attainment of responsible maturity. Further failed attempts contributed to further strains in the relationship, including an extramarital affair and separation, yet the couple had pursued ICSI and IVF rather than try donated sperm as a result to Teranit's refusal to contemplate a nonbiological child. During their separation, Nong had contemplated starting a new relationship to have a child but did not. Her aging body now meant that she could not produce viable ova for use in the ICSI procedure. Her opportunity for a biologically related child was now over; donated ova would now be sought for further attempts. This case study reminds us that men's reproductive experiences and negotiations with their partners are complex and it is not sufficient to reduce their motivations and actions to generalizations. We may discern the workings of patriarchy in his actions and attitudes, but also deep affection towards his wife, his willingness to try to overcome their relationship problems and a recognition of her needs and desire for a child.

Conclusions

Investigation of men's experiences of assisted reproduction from their own point of view is crucial to a full understanding of the impact of these technologies. An almost exclusive focus upon women in many previous studies of assisted reproductive technologies has ignored and further marginalized the involvement of men with infertility treatment and how their attitudes and behaviours affect treatment and the use of these technologies. For Thai men, failure to produce a child can be highly discrediting in a cultural context where fatherhood has traditionally been associated with manhood and fertility with male strength and virility. Despite the prevalence of male factor infertility, men remain marginalized within infertility clinics, which focus attention and interventions upon women. Arbitrary exclusions of men from procedures upon their wives further minimizes their involvement.

More research on men's involvement with assisted reproductive technologies is needed. Because my study was clinic based I was not able to interview men who were unable to accompany their partners to clinic appointments. Thus I have not collected the stories of men whose work commitments prevented them from attending the clinics, nor those who may have been too disinterested to bother or too embarrassed. Further studies need to capture how these absent men relate to the treatments. None of the men or couples in this study admitted to having sexual dysfunctions causing infertility, an underappreciated cause of infertility – this may be because such cases might have been referred to other specialities rather than be treated within infertility clinics that are primarily staffed with gynaecologists. This too would be an important area for further research.

Chapter 6 highlighted the patriarchal relations influencing women's submission to and experience of assisted reproductive technologies. In this chapter it is clear there are pressures upon men as well, both to fulfil their partners' expectations and desires to produce a child, and from societal expectations and their families and male friends. This pressure is also a product of patriarchal views of masculinity linking fertility with virility and maintaining the family line. The infertile man in Thailand is a subject of ridicule for failing to fulfil normative expectations of manhood. Few admit to their infertility but allow the common assumption that infertility is linked to the complexities of women's reproductive system to prevail. Like their female partners, men participate in a process of medicalization of their conditions, having sexual intercourse at appropriate times, producing sperm samples to schedule and in some cases undergoing painful testicular surgeries and extractions in pursuit of a biological child. In this regard they too embody these technologies. This process of medicalization may mitigate the stigma of their infertility, but also subjects them to humiliating experiences and pain. Some appear to avoid the embarrassment and loss of face by maintaining their distance from the clinics as much as possible while financially supporting their wives' efforts; others embrace the medical discourse and are open to discussing their experiences and knowledge of IVF with other men.

Technologies such as ICSI offer new possibilities for even severely infertile men to father a biologically related child but also pose new conundrums for couples. The subsequent chapter will explore the consequences for couples of other technologies such as surrogacy and egg donation.

Notes

1. As Jackson notes, the single Thai term *phet* defies translation as 'sex', 'gender' or 'sexuality'. It crosses a semantic range of what in English are divided between biological, gender, sexuality and sexual intercourse (Jackson and Cook 1999: 4).

2. The emphasis on masculine potency is also seen in traditional cosmology. As Sparkes (1995: 83) notes, female spirits are associated with reproduction and nurturing such as *mae thoranii* (mother earth), *mae phosop* (mother rice) or *mae nam* (mother water). Male nature spirits are active, aggressive and powerful with the ability to activate and protect passive female powers.
3. Comparing the position of physiologically healthy women with that of healthy organ donors, Lorber (1989) questions why doctors do not provide protective mechanisms for women who may not wish to undergo procedures such as would be offered for instance for potential organ donors who may not feel inclined to undertake the risky invasive surgery involved (such as fake medical countra-indications).

Chapter 9

Carrying the Merit

> My eldest sister agreed to be a surrogate mother for me (using my egg and my husband's sperm). I felt as if I was born again. Both my hubby and I were happy. My sister has already got three children. She helped me because she wanted to see me having a complete/perfect family.... It was a bit risky as my sister was already thirty-eight [years old] then. I asked my sister to stop working and let me look after her. I prayed all the time. I just wished to have a baby to make my hubby happy as he really wanted to have a baby.... Then, I learned that my sister was carrying a baby boy. My sister stayed at my place all the time to ensure that this baby is really mine. During the pregnancy, sometimes I was afraid that my baby wouldn't love me or was worried whether he would know that I am his mother.... The first time I saw the baby, I was overwhelmed. My sister breast-fed him for a month. This didn't worry me as she is my sis and she loves the baby, of course. After my sister returned to her family, she still came to help me during the day. Since the baby was born, my family has changed. Now I know what a complete family is. I am so lucky to have a baby and I have my sister to thank for this.

Her sister/surrogate writes: 'She is my youngest sis and I love her a lot. I didn't hesitate to carry a child for her. During pregnancy, I stayed at her place the whole year to ensure that this baby is hers. When my body was ready, the doctor transferred my sister's embryos to my body.... During pregnancy, I felt that I was the baby's birth mother. I loved and bonded to this baby but I also knew that he would stay with his family (my sister). After giving birth, I still helped my sis raise the child and my sis was alright with this. The first word he called me was 'mum' and he called

> my sis 'mama'. He is gentle to me. However, if his mother (my sis) is there too, he will be with her. Sometimes, when I don't see him, I miss him and feel lonely. I love him like I love my own children. My sis and her hubby said that when their son reaches the age of independence, they may tell him that I'm the surrogate mother. Whether they will tell him or not, it doesn't matter to me. I did what I did willingly. My sis still has some embryos left. If she would like to have another child, I am happy to do it again for her. I'm happy to see my sister's family happy. I have received a lot of good things in return for this good deed. I always get what I wish for. Perhaps this is because of this good thing that I have done. I believe that being a surrogate mum is a good deed. That's why it's called 'um bun' [carrying merit / good deeds].'

Accounts of surrogacy in the Thai media and popular press tend to depict overwhelmingly positive arrangements usually between sisters. The quotes above come from a chapter on surrogacy from the educational book with a mixed Thai and English title, *Yak pen mae khae khad jai* Mommy's story' (Threechana and Pimonsing 2004: 203) aimed at infertility patients and the general public. Such images of harmonious surrogacy arrangements are fostered by the medical profession and agencies promoting their surrogacy services. These narratives celebrate the idea of 'warm' family relations so valued in Thailand and Buddhist ideology of women as nurturing altruists. They are fictions in so much as they elide any conflicts, equivocation or stress in the relationship. The image of a shared pregnancy experience and the sharing of care of the child presents an ideal possibility of motherhood as a communal and extended rather than individualized and privatized experience. The surrogate here describes her desire to enrich the family of her sister by way of her body. This included a conscious sharing of the pregnancy with them in such a way as to make them feel like parents during the gestation, framing the experience in terms of a growing relationship in which both women are attached to the child, rather than as a disembodied womb. In turn the sister/surrogate maintains a valued relationship with the child.

In this chapter I explore the relationship between a commissioning parent and her surrogate from the point of view of the commissioning parent. It is based upon a series of interviews with Ying, a woman with a long history of infertility treatment, in which she reveals a little of the experience and emotions during repeated attempts at a surrogate pregnancy. In stark contrast to the account above, it highlights the complexities of the relationship between an intended parent and surrogate. Given that surrogacy remains misunderstood in Thai society, Ying wished for her surrogacy to remain secret, to the extent that we were never introduced to the surrogate, nor did Ying ever intend for any child born to know the full details of the surrogacy. Ying's narrative reflects Thai understandings of motherhood and gender relations but also highlights the hierarchical relationship between surrogate and intended parent. Although initially described as motivated by altruism, the financial arrangements of 300,000 baht (US $10,000) 'compensation' leaves little doubt as to the commercial nature of the relationship. This financial relationship and the proprietal rights it implies over the surrogate's body is a repeated theme in Ying's narrative. While we may empathize with her desire for a child, the objectification evident in her attitude towards her surrogate reveals insidious power differentials.

Not every surrogacy arrangement is as problematic or vexed as the case of Ying, yet it is clear that the lack of support and clear regulations in Thailand at the time made a problematic arrangement even more so. The final part of this chapter looks at the new draft legislation regarding surrogacy and the implications this has for the practice of surrogacy in Thailand as well as Thai concepts of parenthood.

Surrogacy in Thailand

There are two main forms of surrogacy. The first, termed 'traditional', 'partial' or 'genetic surrogacy' is when a woman uses her own ova to be fertilized either through some form of artificial insemination, intercourse or IVF and then carries the resulting pregnancy to birth for other (commissioning or intended) parents. She is the genetic parent of the offspring. In 'gestational' or 'host surrogacy', the surrogate has no genetic relation to the embryos implanted in her womb; she gestates the embryos and gives birth to the child for the intended parents. Although various forms of traditional surrogacy arrangements have long existed, gestational surrogacy and ova donation developed through the growth of assisted reproductive technologies. IVF technologies allowed a range of new possibilities for various forms of gestational surrogacy for people who previously had no opportunity to have genetically related children. Now an infertile couple can use any combination of donated or their own gametes and have the resultant embryo implanted in the womb of a surrogate to carry the pregnancy and give birth to the child. The fact that the gestational surrogate has no genetic relationship to the resultant child made surrogacy more attractive for surrogates and intended parents.

Many countries have struggled to provide timely legislative responses for the rapid technical advances of assisted reproductive technologies. This is certainly true of Thailand which has struggled to regulate the industry in the face of a burgeoning international trade in assisted reproductive services, especially surrogacy. Until recently in Thailand there was no legislation regulating surrogacy. As noted in chapter 1, the Thai Medical Council introduced professional guidelines in 1997 and 2001 for assisted reproductive technologies, including surrogacy (Announcements 1/2540 and 21/2544). These guidelines limited surrogacy to married couples, banned commercial transactions and stated that the surrogate must be a biological relative of the married couple. However, these guidelines had no legislative force and each clinic and hospital was granted discretion with regards to surrogacy arrangements. At the time of this research it was clear that a variety of surrogacy arrangements were being undertaken. The lack of regulation provided little protections for those undertaking surrogacy arrangements, nor for the children born of those arrangements.

Draft legislation contained in the Assisted Reproductive Technologies Bill number 167/2553, was approved by the Thai cabinet in May 2010, passed by the first House of Representatives in 2014 but at the time of writing had not been ratified into law (see chapter 1). This chapter thus captures the realities of surrogacy arrangements during a period of loose regulation. At the time of this study in 2008, surrogates faced an ambiguous position as to their rights, conditions, forms of payment or compensation and protection. Intending parents using surrogates to form a family were faced with a difficult and ambiguous situation in which any contracts had no legal force, and their legal rights over a child produced through surrogacy were unclear. Although posed to change with the new legislation, under section 1546 of the Thai Civil and Commercial Code, the woman who gives birth to a child was regarded as the legal mother of that child. When a child is born to an unwed woman, she alone was recognized as having the legal rights over that child. Under the same Code, the father of a child who was not married to the mother at the time of birth has no parental rights over that child even if recorded on the birth certificate or able to prove his biological parentage.[1] Thus intended parents at the time of this fieldwork had to adopt a child born through surrogacy.

Despite the greater acceptance of assisted reproductive technologies in Thai society, certain procedures such as surrogacy retain an ambivalent status. Yet even surrogacy shows signs of incorporation into Thai notions of reproduction. There has been a gradual change apparent in social attitudes towards surrogacy seen through the language used to describe it. When the term first appeared in newspapers, a range of terms were used from the formal descriptive terms *'tham hay mii luk day doi kanjang khon uen tangkhan'* (having a child through the use of another person to carry the pregnancy) (*Matichon*, 31 May 1987) and *'kan rapjang tangkhan'* (process of hiring a pregnancy) (*Daily News*, 7 August 1987). Such terms are dispassionate descriptions of third-party involvement in reproduction and the use of *'rapjang'* implied the use of hired labour and a commercial relationship. By 2000 the term *'kan rapjang um thong'* (process of hiring to carry a pregnancy) was used for commercial surrogacy, but also the term *'umbun'* (*Thai Post*, 27 May 2000) can be found for surrogacy following its use in a popular television series. By 2004 *'umbun'* was used for all forms of surrogacy (*Khao Sod*, 23 December 2004). Unlike the other terms, *'umbun'* literally means 'carrying the merit'; *'um'* is used when referring to carrying children around and the merit referred to is the Buddhist merit imparted to women when pregnant and in giving birth. As used in the excerpt from 'Mommy's story' above, this term carries overwhelming positive meanings, positioning surrogacy as a selfless meritorious act creating bonds of obligation and goodwill.

However, surrogacy remains a highly sensitive and secretive practice. The events of 2014 involving international surrogacy, such as the 'Baby Gammy' case described in chapter 1, had dual effects within Thailand. On one hand, the case highlighted the practice in Thailand and was the first time surrogates spoke openly in the media about their involvement, motivations and feelings about their surrogate pregnancies and babies. On the other hand, the threat of legal action against women involved in commercial arrangements and closure of clinics and uncertainty over the continuity of their medical care quickly silenced surrogates again.[2]

The new possibilities presented by the advent of gestational surrogacy dramatically confront societies with divisions between genetic, biological and social parenthood and unsettle notions of kinship (Strathern 1992). Through surrogacy, motherhood has been disarticulated into genetic, birth, adoptive and surrogate maternities, with the potential for three mothers to a single child (Ragoné 1994; Thompson 2005). Such challenges to cultural notions of motherhood and fatherhood have met various cultural and legal responses questioning the ethics and means of regulation (van Niekerk and van Zyl 1995; Parks 2010; Donchin 2010).

Feminist responses to surrogacy have centred on issues of the commodification of women's bodies and exploitation in surrogacy arrangements versus notions of reproductive freedom (Berkhout 2008). Marxist and radical feminists describe surrogacy as the ultimate example of patriarchal medicalization, commodification and exploitation of women's bodies, demeaning to motherhood, with some likening the commercial transaction as akin to a form of prostitution or slavery (Corea et al. 1987; Klein 2008; Arditti, Klein and Minden 1984; Dworkin 1983; Rothman 1988, 1989; Raymond 1995). Liberal feminist approaches respect surrogacy as another reproductive choice for women. Often based upon empirical studies with surrogates, they highlight how women involved in the surrogacy process view their bodies, act as agents negotiating the surrogacy and assert positive meanings to the experience of surrogacy (Roberts 1998; Goslinga-Roy 2000; Ragoné 2005; Teman 2001, 2003, 2010).

Empirical accounts suggest that the experience of surrogacy is complex and appears dependent upon the social and legal context in which it takes place, the level of social acceptability, the social and emotional support for all parties and the nature of the contract between the surrogate and commissioning parents. For example, writing of surrogacy within the context of ardently pronatalist Israel, where state-sponsored ARTs are readily available, Elly Teman (2001) argues against depictions of surrogacy as a form of alienated bodily labour, but suggests that women are able to appropriate their medicalization in positive empowering ways. She describes an intense 'hybridised fusion' that occurs between surrogates and intended mothers, creating a sense of shared embodiment of the pregnancy, similar to that described in the account above (2003, 2010).

In other settings, however, authors have noted how surrogacy relationships tend to reproduce class and race hierarchies, especially in contexts where gestational surrogates tend to come from poorer or racially different backgrounds to the commissioning parents (Ragoné 2000). For example, in the United States gestational surrogates tend to be from poorer black and ethnic backgrounds (Roberts 1995). These differentials are particularly marked in international surrogacy arrangements (Pande 2009, 2011; Vora 2010). Writing of an open surrogacy arrangement in the United States, Gillian Goslinga-Roy (2000) analyzes how biogenetic discourses and class ideologies deny the surrogate's attempt to develop an intimate relationship with the commissioning parents who are unable to even comprehend the surrogate as anything other than as a womb. She provides a nuanced analysis of how class and race structure the embodied experience. As clear in Ying's tense discussion of her surrogacy arrangement below she characterizes the surrogate's role and relationship within a privatized discourse of overcoming adversity and self-sacrifice and with an unselfconscious sense of class privilege. The relationship is a vexed one, filled with ambiguity and mistrust, made all the more stressful due the lack of clear guidelines, support or regulations formalizing or protecting the rights of all parties.[3]

Ying

Not long after starting interviews in one public hospital we met Ying. Ying is forty-four years old. She started using IVF seven years ago and joked that she would be the best person for us to interview as she knew everything about every treatment as she had tried them all and knew every clinic. She is a vibrant, loquacious woman, with a cutting sense of humour. She was one of the oldest women we interviewed and her long history of using IVF has equipped her with detailed explanations of the various procedures and protocols used in a variety of clinics. After marrying when she was thirty-four, she travelled to Japan frequently with her senior marketing job for a multinational Japanese firm. She gave up contraception because of the side effects but after two to three years had not become pregnant and so when she was she was thirty-seven she went to see a doctor at a private hospital. Initially, she tried the ovulation method, then IUI and finally started IVF at that same hospital for two years. Similar to other women in this study, she had given up her job to undergo IVF:

> I had to resign because to do this you have to come often [to the clinic] and I would feel bad for my workmates when I had to come as I would have to leave my work with them. My job used to be in marketing, you have to use your brain a lot and so I felt bad for my workmates. Also [then] I thought it wasn't worth it as I would be pregnant and after birth, who would look after my child? And so at that time I thought I would leave my job but I didn't think it would be this difficult.

After no success she decided to change hospitals and went to a public teaching hospital where she underwent IVF and later ICSI.

By then her husband was also having fertility issues due to his age – his sperm were 'no longer strong'. Throughout the interviews she made no further mention of any male infertility factors, but focused upon her infertility.

During her time at the public hospital she did not like that students were involved in her treatment and so changed again to another public hospital and later a private hospital. During that period she underwent a further seven to eight cycles, tried other hospitals and then changed to the current public hospital where we interviewed her. In total she had been a patient at six different clinics and doctors and undergone cycles for the past seven years. As a Sino-Thai, Ying initially wanted to have a boy and as is common in Thai clinics, was using sperm microsorting to sex select for a male child. But now she said she didn't care:

> It doesn't have to be a boy. My husband would prefer a boy but in the end, whatever. Girl or boy, whatever, it is so long now, we don't care to choose now. As long as the child isn't gay! At first I was choosy, I was doing sex selection all along, but this time I didn't choose. If it was my eggs I selected for sex but now I don't want to choose it is a sad story because it is so long now and the drugs are expensive.

She has started using donated eggs recently. Her aging body and history of multiple treatments meant it was more and more difficult to stimulate ova production and her endometrial lining was thinning, making implantation unlikely. At first she used the eggs of a friend who lives in Los Angeles. 'She flew here to collect eggs, but she was quite old and the Doctor said she was too old at thirty-five and had only ten to twelve eggs.' After no success with those she began using the eggs from the present donor. Ying claimed that young women were coming to clinics to sell their eggs: 'If you go to [a public hospital] and if you don't dress like this and sit among patients then you know some of them come to the hospital to sell eggs … that group knows the right place to sell their eggs, I used to be a patient of Mor X, he was my first doctor. He said, "Go and buy, there are people who sell eggs, just get someone who looks like you."'[4]

Across her seven years of treatment she has had one pregnancy which miscarried at eight weeks. 'I was sad but now I'm not as I think, "OK, if I am pregnant [literally, it sticks] the child will be born or if we have merit [*bun*] and it is born as our child we will be happy to nurture it to be a good member of society. But if we can't then it is nothing because *Phra Jao* [God] has helped us up to this point [to try].” We have done the best we can already. I don’t blame anyone. The story of my treatment is longer than that of other people.’

Apart from her treatment at the infertility clinic she took Chinese medicines, and had undergone acupuncture to stimulate her womb. She had also visited Luang Phor Sathorn (see chapter 3), temples in Ayuttaya and a temple in Singhburi as well as travelling to China to *Jao Mae Kuan Im* at Kuiling to ask for a child. She also gives alms to increase her merit: ‘Every Saturday I give alms to ten monks, all types of food. I make it myself, I don’t buy it! I also give alms to three or seven monks every day.’ Despite all her efforts, she made the extraordinary claim that she did not want a child but was undertaking all the treatment for her husband’s sake. She declared:

> My husband is happy with what I have done up to now. I am doing it for him especially because I don’t want a child. I’m a pessimist, I feel that the world is getting hotter, the economy isn’t good. The exchange rate is bad. I see all is chaotic. If a child is born they have to fight to live. Therefore, *Thep Phra Jao* has said it is good not to have a child as we wouldn’t have any worries. I think like this, but my husband disagrees.... Yes, he really wants one, and I love him a lot because he is a good person. Not that I boast, my husband graduated with a Masters from Chulalongkorn [a prestigious university], he doesn’t drink, he doesn’t smoke, he has never cheated on me, he hasn’t got a girlfriend at work, he returns home for dinner, he is a good man. On the weekends he doesn’t go anywhere and so OK I see he is a good person and so I [accept] the pain and I try for him.

Ying offered to find a woman as a *mia noi* (‘minor wife’) to produce a child for her husband: ‘I would find a *mia noi* for my husband. I would give them a house and do everything. If my husband wanted it I would do it but he doesn’t want it. If my husband agreed with the idea I think the brideprice[5] would be less than the money I spent on hospital fees right?’

While not legal marriages, the practice of having a concubine or minor wife is socially acknowledged in Thai society, particularly among men wealthy enough to support them. The term ‘*mia noi*’ indicates a more permanent relationship than that of mistress, and it is generally expected that wealthy or powerful men will support and maintain one or more *mia noi* as a demonstration of virile masculinity. Producing an heir through a second wife would have been a long-held practice for wealthy and high-status infertile couples in Thailand in the past when polygamy was widely practiced and legal in Thailand. Today, however, women fear their husbands taking on minor wives. As described in chapter 6, infertile women particularly feel vulnerable to desertion by their husband for another woman. Ying here subverts that fear by embracing it as a pragmatic solution to their childlessness. She jokes that the financial costs of arranging and maintaining a *mia noi* could be far cheaper than IVF treatment. Her offer marks her willingness to sacrifice herself for the sake of her husband's fulfilment. The fact that her husband rejected her offer to find a *mia noi* reinforces her discourse of him as a 'good man'.

Throughout her narrative Ying evoked an image of herself as undergoing a persistent struggle against adversity. She contrasted the lack of effort required of fertile couples to have children with that required by those with fertility problems. Her quest involved sacrifice especially for her husband's happiness. The extent of sacrifice is underlined by her offer to find a *mia noi* for her husband. In this way she juxtaposes 'normal' marriage and gender relations – i.e. a wife supplies an heir and tries to keep a husband from having affairs – to her inability to supply an heir and offer of supplying a *mia noi*. These juxtapositions however only serve to underline both her and her husband's virtue in the face of adversity; her willingness to do 'whatever it takes' to supply an heir and his refusal to take on a *mia noi* but remain faithful to her.

> If you have a baby it is OK you can raise a baby, but if you don't have, you have to struggle just to have a baby. Like me I am struggling, struggling. I used to ask him [my husband] would he be OK if I got him a new wife, what kind of wife would he like; doctor, nurse, whatever, I can find one for him, or does he want me to walk out of his life completely? Because I have quite a few houses. Would he like me to go out of his life and ask this lady to live in the house? And he said he didn't want that. I could do that for his happiness. It wouldn't be too much to do. I'm this old now I could stay at the temple, meditating. It's like we have learned a lot in life knowing what life really is about but I see that he is a good man and when he wants to have one [a child], his parents want to have one so I do it. So even the Gods and angels couldn't accuse me of not having tried my utmost. I have dedicated myself to this. But if you ask people in medicine they don't like it because they say if you can't conceive naturally it's OK, no need to try this hard. It is like the higher powers have already determined who will have a child so no need to struggle because having a baby, it is said that it depends on whether your [*phook duang*] horoscope is favourable [*sang bun sang kaam*]. We create merit and demerit in our past lives and then a baby is born joined in our karma [*khu kaam*] in order to pay our debts. Therefore they say it is good that I don't have a baby so I can be a person without a

> karma [i.e. break the cycle of karma as if there is no baby no one will create further karma].

Here Ying suggests she has been advised by doctors not to continue in her quest, to accept her childlessness. She refers to the widespread understandings of predestined fate exhibited in one's horoscope and the karmic notion that children and parents have been linked in some form in past incarnations; hence they continue to have lives that are intertwined until their karmic cycle is broken. This is used by some Buddhist commentators (and referred to by doctors) as a means of accepting one's infertility as a positive karmic outcome, indicating that one has completed the karmic cycle and thus is not condemned to repeating the cycle – rather, they are a step closer to removing the ties to the material world and achieving nirvana.

Ying has tried donated eggs for several cycles without success and at the time of our interview her 25-year-old egg donor was going to act as a surrogate as well. They were undergoing cycles together, being implanted with embryos at the same time in the hope that one of them would achieve a pregnancy. In our first interview she described the surrogate as 'like a niece, what is she, she's a friend but not someone close to me at all'. In using the term 'niece' she was using a fictive kin term, indicating someone younger than herself, not a family member. But she was coy about providing any further details. She did reveal that she has known her surrogate for five years and explained the criteria for choosing a surrogate:

> She is young, only twenty-five years old and has a baby already, her child is two years and a half and she has similar face and skin colour similar to me so OK. And one more thing, if she is young, in my opinion she is more likely to get pregnant easily and also when someone has already given birth, it's like their uterus lining has been cleaned and the uterus is clean and it will be easier to implant.

We asked Ying how this woman came to be a surrogate:

> She said OK because she has seen me trying for so long and she is a person who is open-minded, and she is sympathetic. She saw that I go to the hospital often and wondered if she might be able to help. If she could she would. And she said that if she could help she would make merit [through this act] to give life to a person is something which grants a lot of merit. So she is happy to help. It isn't easy to find someone like this because they have to be pregnant for nine months, if they are not sincere they won't do it. But she is sympathetic.... At first she [just gave eggs] for me to carry. But I have being doing it for

> a long time now and the [my endometrial] lining is not thick enough now. So now she is prepared to carry it [a pregnancy] herself.

It took a year between her initial talks with the surrogate to commencing treatment, 'because her child was still small and was breastfeeding'. She did not intend to tell any future child about their origins: 'When they are big already I will tell them some things. If they accept it. But when they are twenty and adolescent I couldn't tell them as they are unstable emotionally and can't accept it. … I'm not sure.' When we asked Ying how she felt about using a surrogate, she revealed her fears that the surrogate might decide to keep the baby:

> If she gives birth I will accept it [the child] because not many people know [about the surrogacy] right? And the surrogate will not keep the baby. However, I am prepared for both best and worst case scenarios. I talked to my husband. There is so much news that most surrogates when they are pregnant they tend to have a bond and don't hand the baby over. If it happens that she won't hand over the baby I have decided to let her keep the baby. She would have to bring the child up and not hand the baby over to us. Because I am not a bad woman but I don't want to have any moral problems. [I don't want] a child to be passed back and forth between us [when it is big]. This person is very important. She has to be someone who is screened well. First if she has her own child already she is less likely to want to keep the child, right? Secondly, she needs to be someone who wants to make money. She needs money to pay for her household expenses because her mother is a farmer. The majority of [surrogates] prefer the money from us rather than the child.

As noted above, at the time of the interview, under Thai laws the woman who gave birth to a child was registered at the mother on a birth certificate. Contracting parents would have to adopt the child born as a result of surrogacy and surrogacy contracts were legally unenforceable. When we asked Ying about this she suggested that she would 'have to chat with the doctor about this a little'. 'I have had treatment with the doctor and the doctor had introduced this method to us and helped us halfway so I will ask the doctor to help us a little bit more' by falsifying the name of the mother on the birth certificate. She claimed she had had a friend for whom this was done at a regional hospital to avoid a child growing up believing they were adopted. She had promised to pay the surrogate 300,000 baht (US $10,000) for the surrogacy as well as her medical expenses.

Her relationship with the surrogate was underscored with mistrust about what she described as the 'power' of the surrogate:

> If she gets pregnant then we will draft a contract. I am thinking about how to write it to make it sound soft. Because if we make it sound like a 'contract' it will be too rigid and against [*manusiyatham*] morals/ethics. I am scared because I have to make a contract for me to be comfortable but even if we make one we can't enforce it because it is not my eggs. If it was a court case I would lose. As I said I told her because she watches TV and there was news about surrogates who refuse to hand over the baby and I told her that I wouldn't accept that, that it she wants to raise the child she can have it. A child is not like gold, it [man] is a person and so I'd let it go. I wouldn't pay. It is like we have spoken already that I wouldn't pay if she kept the child. When I take her to the clinic twenty per cent of patients are wealthy. The surrogate's mother sees that there are a lot of unsuccessful cases and she can see the power of her position.

The couple remained secretive about their use of a surrogate. Their family on both sides knew about the IVF treatment but not surrogacy:

> They don't know. They know that I come for treatment but they don't know which method I'm using. They don't need to know. They may not accept it. And in addition, they are in [another province], they live a long way away so they don't have a chance to know. And again they never come so we would keep doing this for eight or nine months and then say 'I've given birth'. My side they don't recommend my treatment at all, because I came from a tough background. At my house there were eight girls and one boy. Only a few got married and so they say, 'She has encountered economic problems and now is comfortable so why should she make it difficult for herself now?' They don't support me in this.

Ying carefully supervised her surrogate, driving her to and from clinic appointments and supplementing her food:

> I supervise her diet often and visit her regularly. I'm very tired. I drive each day four times from my house to hers then to the hospital and then from the hospital to her house and then to mine. I am the most tired! On the days when she has to bring her child along I am very tired because her child is naughty, has to be watched all the time and eats a lot and vomits. I have to wipe up after the child's wee and poo, all the time, I'm tired. And I'm not only coming one day. Four times for ultrasounds, I have to look after the child.

At first Ying's case seemed like so many other women we interviewed, albeit she had a longer history of treatment and was far more open in discussing the use of a surrogate. Nevertheless, the more we spoke with her, the complexity of her feelings and quest for a child became more apparent. Two and a half months later in a further interview with Ying she described how things had not gone well with the surrogate. Firstly, the young woman had suffered ovarian hyperstimulation syndrome (OHSS), a life-threatening condition.

> After the stimulation she had plenty of eggs creating the side effect which was fluid retention [ovarian hyperstimulation]. The doctor explained to me that within one egg the water is equivalent to one glass of water and she had too many eggs, an abnormal number. Normally people get fourteen or thirteen. But the surrogate mother had forty-two.... I consider that I'm lucky that I have found her. If this happened to other people I might be sued right? Because it was swollen so she couldn't sleep like it was rising up at night so she had to sit still for two or three days.... She couldn't lie down and she didn't tell me about this and the doctor said this might have killed her. She is very patient. She is doing this for me so she is patient she looked like a panda bear with black eyes. She couldn't sleep during the day or at night but I think she had been given too much stimulation drug so this makes the eggs incomplete. Because too much drug has been absorbed by the eggs.

Despite this setback, the cycle continued.

> The doctor expected a successful result, he went to the max. Put them [the embryos] in to get twins, even though the surrogate mother is quite small her womb is perfect. But after fifteen days she went mountain climbing because she is young and energetic so she climbed up a tree and up a cliff so I'm not so sure whether it happened because of this. So this resulted in either the chromosome or the implantation didn't take place and it turned out to be a sack of water, no heart, It is like the white egg turns to be a placenta and the egg yolk didn't turn to be a human. If we leave it longer it will turn to be a *khai khaw* [incomplete white egg with partially formed embryo referring to a chicken egg with partly formed chick]. I have seen that before I have experienced that myself so I decided that in the fifth or sixth week because people who had embryo transfer a week later than her at eight weeks you could see the heart beating but in her case there is no heart beating so I decided to abort. So the doctor gave a suppository medicine.... In her case it was only five to six weeks so it had nothing it came out as two or three lumps of blood, like caviar. Round caviar, two or three eggs. Before that lump came out she told me she

> had a stomach ache but the doctor told her previously that after she put in the suppository drug that it would feel like she was having a period and she acknowledged that. It's good that she is rather patient.

Ying decided to try the next cycle herself, so she underwent a curettage and took hormones to stimulate the production of her endometrium to try yet another cycle with donated ova:

> I'm afraid that when you hire [*jang*] someone they promise everything but we don't monitor her all the time so we didn't know that after the implantation they will look after themselves as good as we do. In addition, my experience of the first time with her makes me feel that I'm taking a lot of risk because the cost of each cycle is high so for the time being we are leaving a question mark but haven't abandoned it completely. So I will stimulate myself first and told the doctor to do whatever it takes to have them put the embryo in me to finish it. This is because sometimes the consequences [of surrogacy] are too problematic. I have to be the one who sings and dances by myself. I will be very tired. Because I haven't had a child yet. If I had a child and I was tired then it would be worth it. But I am tired but without a baby. I have to look after her four or five o'clock in the morning: pick her up pick her kid up. It's like sometimes I wonder if she feels I'm her slave. So this is tiring. And when I ask her [*man*] to look after herself. Just to have this duty she didn't do it as I wanted her to. I went all the way to the pier to buy fish for her 1,000 baht each and I carried the fish to her [man] and I didn't know whether she ate it or not whether her baby or her husband ate it. I don't want to be narrow-minded but I am tired I can't stop myself from thinking because I have done everything by myself. So this time I came to stimulate the lining again.

In this narrative of the unsuccessful first cycle with the surrogate, Ying vents her frustration at the tiring process of IVF and surrogacy. Significantly, through the use of pronouns, in Thai she transforms the surrogate from a 'young niece' to the word '*man*' ('it'), a pronoun usually reserved for nonhuman objects or animals. This literal denial of subjectivity both indicates her frustration and anger at the surrogate for failing in her view to take appropriate caution following implantation as though that were the reason for the failure of the cycle, even though she indicates that there were possibly chromosomal reasons or some other issue with implantation. Such objectification of the surrogate also occurs in the clear statement that it is Ying's decision whether to stimulate the surrogate for a further cycle, with no reference to the surrogate herself or acknowledgement of the medical risks of this following her experience of OHSS. She clearly talks of her as hired labour (using the term *'jang'*) and resents the effort she has undertaken, 'like a slave', to feed the surrogate good food like fish, arrange for her to attend medical appointments and provide childcare while she does so. In exchange, she speaks of the surrogate's duty and failure to 'look after herself' following implantation and the subsequent need to monitor the surrogate closely. Throughout, embryos, wombs and bodies are described as expensive commodities for manipulation, surveillance, monitoring and maintenance. Throughout she makes a statement of the physical, emotional and phenomenological effort of continuing treatment herself, expressed through the metaphor of 'tiredness' of her body. But as she notes with irony, this tiredness is not as a result of pregnancy, not of actual motherhood, but of the effort to become one.

Ying's response to the failure of the first cycle was to initiate a further cycle in which the remaining embryos were transferred to herself. Her relationship with the surrogate had clearly deteriorated and the description of the surrogate as 'open-minded and sympathetic' in the interview two months earlier had now become one of 'those types of people' who was acquisitive and manipulative, making constant demands for money.

> It looks as if when you are too friendly with this type of people they may not be *krengjai* towards us. Because she keeps asking for reimbursement and I open my purse, open my purse, 10,000, 2000, 3000. Suppose the baby is delivered and you can see its face and eyes, what will I do next? She might squeeze us [for more money], what will we do? Will we kill the baby? We won't do that right? So during this time she hasn't had her [period] yet so I stimulate myself once or twice.

The concept of *krengjai* (deferential heart) she evokes here refers to a Thai notion of showing respect, politeness and consideration to another person, particularly to a superior. It is the art of not putting another person in a difficult situation or making them lose face. A failure to display appropriate *krengjai* suggests poor manners, a lack of appropriate sentiment and a failure of knowing one's place.

Ying feared that the surrogate would continue to ask for money in subsequent years even after a birth. With no legal protection for surrogacy arrangements she evoked an image of a continuous blackmailing from the surrogate for money other than the agreed fee of 300,000 baht.

> What she is doing this for? I know she is doing it for the money as a first priority. Suppose it doesn't work and suppose we keep doing this she will get money from me every month, this is something she

can demand from me. So it tends to be indefinite, right? But for us this is like our loss. And it is mentally exhausting also.... No matter what, we're going to be disadvantaged no matter what. If this became a court case we would be disadvantaged anyway. We will always lose giving me even more depression.

She suggested the surrogate would continue to ask for money because she is lower class: 'It will be like this because they are not middle class they are lower class. They work in the morning and eat at night.' Yet even while she is commodifying the surrogate's services, she also described the financial motivation as a sign of the surrogate's lower nature or class. This is in marked contrast to her own portrayals of her motivation earlier as purely unselfish (for her husband's happiness). She noted that even a failed cycle still resulted in financial gain for the surrogate, as though the surrogate might deliberately undermine the success of the surrogacy as evidenced by her failing to undertake a prolonged period of bed rest following embryo transfer.

Unlike other people she knew who had used surrogacy services, Ying claimed that she was not very restrictive and painted a picture of other contracting parents policing all aspects of their surrogates' lives, even toileting. Her surveillance of her surrogate she insisted was minimal:

I'm not like others. In the case of my friend, the surrogate mother couldn't do a thing. 'Lie down! Lie down!' And when the surrogate walked down the stairs. 'Where are you going?' And gave her a potty. She hired a nurse to look after the surrogate if she wanted to pee or poo they would give a potty. Whereas I am more lenient. If she wanted to climb stairs then that's OK. I don't want her to be stressed as stress is not good to force her to do something that is silly. She could go wherever she wanted but I just asked for her not to ride a motorcycle, don't run up the stairs, just these little things and in terms of food we supplied her all, no matter if it was medicine, vitamins, supplementary foods. I even looked after her kid and sometimes I was bored. A child of that age is really a pain.... I explained to her that I am not like other contracting mothers. If it was another person hiring her they would only let her lie down. But here you can do what you like, go where you want, only thing you can't do is run up the stairs, no running and the important thing is she has a motorcycle and she shouldn't ride it, that's all.

In a final twist in her narrative, Ying described an informal 'adoption' that she had tried seven years earlier before her IVF treatment. She started to raise a baby from local rubbish collectors:

> They were going to leave the baby with the orphanage and I didn't know that they used to leave the baby with the orphanage before and it is not the huge orphanage of Thammasat, just an orphanage in a community where they look after kids and they have missionaries looking after this orphanage. And these missionaries look after these kind of kids, around twenty to thirty [kids]. And I don't know what happened to her [the mother], she didn't want to raise the kid anymore and she saw me being wealthy and so she left the baby with me and so, 'Ok I'll raise the child.'

The mother took the child away from the orphanage and then left the baby with Ying to raise. She cared for the baby for two to three months.

> After I looked after the kid for a while the orphanage was panicking because she didn't let them know. So the people from the orphanage came to see why I raised the child.... I felt annoyed. When the child grew, because the child grew up very quickly, the parents came and asked for money and when the child grew we had to take him to see the doctor because the baby was not complete [disabled]. The baby had no anus so they had to make a hole. That required surgery. So I couldn't bear it. So I gave it back to the missionaries. If this kept happening the parents would just keep coming and when the child grows up the parents would just keep coming in the morning, in the evening, I would be out of my mind and what would I get in the end? I would have to tell the child I am not their parent and the child may return to their parents so while the child is still young better to give it back.

As a result of this failed informal adoption, Ying vowed never to adopt a child but would prefer to remain childless. Her description of her experience with adoption upholds the cultural ideology of the biological child so central to assisted reproductive technologies (Becker 2000: 132) and to her Sino-Thai background. Her fear of financial demands, and of losing the child to its biological parents is evident. Informal adoptions occur in Thailand, usually between family members; this one seems to have occurred under somewhat dubious circumstances and it is unclear what arrangements were made between the parents and Ying who glossed over details.

At a further follow-up phone call, Ying explained that following the failure of her attempt at implantation the surrogate underwent a further cycle which again failed. She felt frustrated and depressed. At that time she explained that she knew of three other couples trying surrogacy; one couple had achieved a pregnancy with their surrogate who was their house servant, while another couple had a three-month-old baby. Six months later when we rang her again, her surrogate was pregnant on her third attempt, and in 2008 she delivered a healthy baby boy.

'Delicate Matters': The New Draft Legislation and Surrogacy in Thailand

As noted in chapter 1, the need for legislation to regulate assisted reproductive practice in Thailand was suggested as early as 1987. The broad public became aware of surrogacy when it hit the headlines in 1988 with the much-publicized case of a famous actress, 'Mayura', who was said to be considering using her sister as a surrogate to carry a child. The public reaction at the time was so outraged that she later denied such plans.[6] Although the Thai Medical Council introduced professional guidelines in 1997 and 2001 for assisted reproductive technologies, including surrogacy, these lack legal force and, as evident in Ying's case, surrogacy practice has not always been undertaken in accordance to the recommendations.

Reports of the imminent development of the new draft legislation on assisted reproductive technologies continued in 2001 and 2004 and often focused upon the need to regulate surrogacy.[7] In 2004 at a seminar on surrogacy law held by the Ministry of Social Development and Human Security, the 'Father of IVF' in Thailand, Dr Pramuan, was quoted as stating that the demand for surrogacy was increasing and that over twenty surrogate pregnancies had already occurred in specialist hospitals mostly to multimillionnaires.[8] Media depictions of surrogacy were largely supportive of the need for legislation. For example, the weekly magazine *Woman Plus* sympathetically related the plight of three women who required surrogates or ova donation to introduce a discussion of the new draft legislation.[9] It suggested that 'the technology has gone so far and these are delicate matters but our laws are still behind'. However, the bill was slow in coming to cabinet due in part to the political instability during this period. The draft Assisted Reproductive Technologies Bill 167/2553 was approved by the Thai cabinet in May 2010 yet proceeded no further following repeated government instability. A military coup d' état took place on 22 May, 2014 introducing military rule to Thailand. The military government acted to shut down the international surrogacy trade following the events throughout 2014: the Baby Gammy case, the case of the Japanese business man who had hired multiple surrogates and other revelations of infringements of the Thai medical guidelines. The House of Representatives passed the legislation in 2015 and the legislation was expected to be promulgated sometime in 2015, 28 years since the first calls for regulation (see chapter 1).

Although details of the final draft of the legislation were not fully public at time of writing, it was expected that the new Assisted Reproductive Technologies Bill will set a number of conditions on surrogacy that largely follow the original draft from 2010. Under the legislation a surrogate mother must have given birth to a child already and, if married, her husband must consent to the surrogacy. Surrogates must be related to the intending parents, although not a parent or daughter of either of the intending parents, effectively removing any chance of surrogacy for couples without appropriate female relatives. Only Thai married heterosexual couples would be considered eligible for surrogacy arrangements. The Bill prohibits the surrogate from also being an egg donor in the surrogacy. Commercial surrogacy is not permitted (Section 23), and the terms of the surrogacy, payment of the costs and expenses of the surrogate mother and the conditions of the surrogacy are to be determined by a third regulatory body (yet to be determined, possibly the Medical Council or University hospital) with the approval of the Child Protection Committee (Section 24). In addition, the bill has consequences for the 'medical facilitation' companies that have operated in Thailand for foreign couples, as Section 25 of the Bill makes it an offence to act as an intermediary or broker for surrogacy arrangements or to accept financial or other benefits for the engagement or management of surrogacy. Section 26 also prohibits advertisements seeking women wishing to act as surrogates whether for commercial purposes or otherwise.

Significantly for intending parents, Section 27 of the draft surrogacy law removes the ambiguity over the parentage of a child born of surrogacy arrangements. It provides that a child born through means permitted under the Assisted Reproductive Technologies Act will be deemed to be the legitimate child of the commissioning parents, not the surrogate or other person who provided genetic material. This fundamentally changes the legal definition of motherhood from the birthing mother to privilege those who have commissioned the birth, reversing long-standing cultural and legal traditions that define kinship through gestation.[10]

Under such laws, the arrangement Ying had with her surrogate would be illegal, although it remains to be seen what level of 'compensation' will be paid to surrogates under the new laws. Under these laws the question of who would be named on the birth certificate as parents would be resolved as the intending parents' rights are recognized in this legislation and there would be no legal need to adopt a child born through a surrogacy arrangement. As noted in chapter 1, the delays in regulating medically assisted reproductive technologies is partly due to a failure of legislators to keep up with the rapidly changing technologies, but there has also been little incentive to regulate within the highly profitable intimate industry of IVF in Thailand. In particular, the practice of surrogacy has largely remained highly secretive. The very fact that this legislation exists now speaks of how surrogacy is becoming much more common. Thai society has been forced to consider whether and in what forms surrogacy is to be accepted and what will be the appropriate ethical framework and protections for those involved. Once the legislation is finally debated in parliament and ratified, it remains to be seen what changes will ensue in practice and what effects this will have upon surrogacy in Thailand.

Conclusions

Surrogacy challenges Thai definitions of motherhood. Until the recent legislation, definitions of Thai motherhood have been uterocentric – embedded in beliefs about the importance of gestation and birth as a marker of a woman's adult status and Buddhist ideology which lauds the pains and sacrifices of pregnancy and birth as meritorious. The sufferings of pregnancy and birth have been understood to build emotional bonds and obligations between mother and child, *bun khun* relationships which result in a debt of gratitude between a child and its mother. Such understandings of motherhood and its relation to the sacrifices of pregnancy are reinforced by most methods of assisted reproduction in which women undertake extraordinary efforts and suffering to become pregnant. However, surrogacy challenges such understandings of motherhood and as such has remained less accepted in Thai society than other forms of assisted reproduction. New forms of parenthood and relatedness are now to be legally recognized, in which the intention to be the 'social' parent takes primacy. In the case of those using donor eggs and sperm, it poses new forms of making kinship without genetics. It challenges Thai society to rethink relationships which were formerly naturalized.

Understanding the complexities of assisted reproductive technologies requires attention to the lives of individuals most affected by these technologies and how their hopes and fears interact within the specific cultural and socioeconomic context. As this chapter notes, in the absence of clear regulations, individuals like Ying were left unaided to negotiate surrogacy arrangements and the new forms of relatedness they entail. Her narrative demonstrates the complex movements between gratitude and mistrust, fears of financial blackmail and a sense of class privilege that permeated her relationship with her surrogate. The surrogate herself was gradually reduced across the narrative from an altruistic, generous and patient individual to an object hired for the nine months of the pregnancy who was to be monitored and later elided from the child's biography. Although it is clear that the power differential was in her favour as a wealthy woman of high social status, Ying herself spoke of the power of the surrogate to demand money, support and childcare, presenting herself as the exploited party. The voice of the surrogate is absent, silenced by the power relations that define their relationship. The narrative works as a cautionary tale, that in stark contrast to the romantic images of blissful surrogacy to be found in clinic advertising and the popular press, the lived experience of surrogacy may fall far short of these ideals and 'carrying merit' may be another means for the subordination of women by other (wealthy) women.

Notes

1. These provisions derive from reforms of the Thai legal code that occurred in the reign of King Vajiravudh in the early twentieth century which attempted to create a standardized family structure to ensure consistency in inheritance, parentage and divorce. Influenced heavily by Western laws, the reforms outlawed polygyny and set heterosexual monogamy as the Thai legal marital standard. Hence children born out of marriage were legally defined as their (disreputable) mother's child with no legal recognition of their male parentage (Loos 1999).
2. Although I do not address Thailand's international reproductive and surrogacy trade in this book, I have described it elsewhere (Whittaker 2010, 2011, 2012).
3. In presenting this I am mindful of the fact that presenting only one side of the relationship contributes to the objectification of the surrogate and fails to adequately account for her agency in a way that mirrors Ying's own movement through this narrative from acknowledging her surrogate's role to resenting it and objectifying her in her speech.
4. I later asked a doctor at the public hospital she named whether eggs were available for sale by donors at the hospital. He claimed this was false, although such sales may have happened in the past.

5. 'Brideprice' refers to the money paid by a husband's family to the wife's family upon marriage which is customary in Thailand.
6. *Daily News*, 28 September 1988, 'Nu Tuk is discouraged about *phasom tiam*'.
7. *Matichon*, 8 July 2001, 'Pushing surrogate baby legislation, problems with rights, concerns over complicated future'.
8. *Thai Rath*, 23 December 2004, 'พม. หนุนออกกฎหมายเด็ก อุ้มบุญ' (Ministry of Social Development and Human Security supports surrogacy legislation introduction). *KhaoSod*, 23 December 2004, 'ถก 'พรบ. อุ้มบุญ' กันวุ่น-แย่งเด็ก : แฉเศรษฐีถึง 20 รายแห่ทำกันแล้ว' (Discussion on surrogacy law – competing for baby. 20 millionaires have used surrogacy).
9. *Woman Plus*, 2006, 'Following the surrogacy law'. http://women.sanook.com/mom-baby/knowledge/lifestyle_24606.php (retrieved 10 November 2006). This article followed controversy after a public seminar by the Thai Medical Council entitled, 'What society thinks about egg sperm and embryo trade?' which revealed the commercial trade in gametes in a number of hospitals in Thailand. The president of medical ethics from the Medical Association of Thailand stated, 'This kind of trade is like abortion which is available every day and everywhere although it's illegal.' Although the Medical Council insisted that gametes could not be traded, only donated (*'borijak'*), it was suggested that 'greedy' women do sell their eggs. Again the spectre of becoming 'like the US where they trade openly [in ova and sperm]' was raised. *Thai Rath*, 31 October 2001, 'Beware of danger. Females sell eggs, males sell sperms. Openly trade at many hospitals. Foreigners rush to buy!' *Matichon*, 31 October 2001, ดาราหนุนซื้อขายไข่ – อสุจิ แนวโน้มอนาคตธุรกิจเฟื่อง (Celebrities support egg/sperm trade, likely to be a promising business in the future). *Thai Rath*, 2 November 2001, 'Five famous hospitals trading eggs and sperms'.
10. This may be contrasted with the situation in Vietnam, where legitimate and legally recognized motherhood remains restricted to birthing mothers and defines surrogacy as illegal, expressly protecting the relatedness between a mother and the children she bears. This derives from deep-seated understandings of the importance of maternal kinship ties (Pashigian 2009).

CONCLUSION

I began this book with a story of an encounter in a lift between a woman undergoing IVF and a woman embracing her newborn baby – an encounter in which what is defined as 'natural' was at stake. Yet in reality, reproduction is far from a 'natural' event, but a highly cultured one, mediated by social rules, gendered expectations and a range of technical interventions. This book charts some of the contradictory positions women face in interventions into reproduction, in this case the use of assisted reproductive technologies. I seek to capture the multiple, productive and sometimes exploitative relationships between technoscience, the medical profession, individual histories and relationships and broader political and economic trends. Writing about assisted reproduction poses challenges for researchers, forcing us to recognize that the aspirations of women and men and enactment of their reproductive rights to access technologies to form families may involve contradictions, opposing moral economies, risks and negative effects. It would be wrong to argue that my book is for or against the use of assisted reproduction; rather, what I have been concerned with is providing insight into how technoscientific interventions into reproduction are manifested in a particular cultural setting and the contradictory effects this has on women and men's lives.

An important insight of science and technology studies is that rather than neutral and objective, technoscience is both reinforced and permeated with the worldviews, desires, fears and values of the society in which it is generated (Harding 1991: ix). Reproductive technologies such as contraception, abortion and infertility treatments are crucial sites for understanding new ideas and imaginaries about nature, gender, kinship and parenthood. Each society grapples with these issues in different ways and in this book the study of assisted reproduction in Thailand provides insight into how Thai understandings of the body and reproduction, gender relations, ethics, religion, politics, kinship, race and nation are entangled in efforts to reproduce. The book title, *Thai in Vitro,* reflects the desire to observe what is distinctly Thai about assisted reproduction in Thailand. The technologies manipulate Thai genetic material, but are also influenced by and reflect particularly Thai values and practices.

Although I draw upon the insights of science and technology studies and cultural studies of globalization, this book may also be read as a methodological assertion of the importance of fieldwork and concepts of culture within a study of a local manifestation of global technoscience. Bruce Kapferer (2000: 189) argues that fieldwork is a means through which anthropologists disrupt taken-for-granted assumptions about practices in lived realities and is vital to the production of empirically generated and critically directed analysis. This is not just in exotic village locales, but, as in this case, within the clinics and hospitals of global urban cities. By tracing the history, context and forms in which IVF is practiced, experienced and thought about by infertile couples, I show the relevance of anthropological approaches to contemporary realities. Not only does this book describe the cultural difference entailed in Thai IVF, but what Kapferer (2000: 186) describes as a central problematic of the discipline, namely, how 'cultural forces are intimate with the direction and shape of human social and political practice'.

In this book I charted the growth of the new intimate industry of reproductive medicine in Thailand. The history of assisted reproduction in Thailand is one of keenness and competition with Asian neighbours for the demonstration of scientific ascendancy to growing concerns over potential excesses. Assisted reproductive technologies have become the centre of a neoliberal assemblage of technologies, skills, pharmaceuticals, cells, bodies and capital which draw upon and create new forms of 'intimate labour' (Boris and Parrenas 2010). The technologies are embedded within networks of personal care relations and affect, they shape the relations between patients and medical staff. The forms of intimate labour carried out within infertility clinics are also being transformed; elsewhere I describe how global mobilities encouraged the development of a trade in reproductive ova and surrogacy services in Thailand (Whittaker 2011, 2012).

The growth of the intimate industry of reproduction has also reinforced economic systems of inequality. The increased privatization of medicine and health care within Thailand allows for the high-tech investments required for this industry to flourish. The effects of capitalist relations runs throughout this book; from the global maldistribution and stratification of access to infertility treatments which favour the wealthy, the commodification of treatment and privatization of clinics, through to the commercialization (and international market) of reproductive services such as surrogacy. The promise and excitement that embraced these technologies in Thailand in the 1990s has been tempered by the visibility of the negative effects of ruthless market forces. The Thai medical profession and regulators have recognized the need for protections for all concerned within the industry; what remains to be seen is whether attempts to regulate the industry will be enforceable.

New biosocial groupings have formed around infertility and the use of reproductive technologies in cyberspace. On the whole these operate complementary to biomedical expertise rather than in opposition to it, but they do allow new forms of self-expression, self-education, criticism and collective identity. Above all, however, such sites tend to maintain the ethos of hope that surrounds assisted reproductive technologies (Franklin 1997). The maintenance of hope and faith despite the numerous setbacks involved in treatment is rigorously promoted in clinics, websites and by staff. As aspects of life and the intimacies of reproduction once placed on the side of fate and karma now become subjects of decisions and intervention, patients are urged to embrace regimes of the self in which they manage their bodies, observe prudent dietary and sexual advice, undertake helpful spiritual practices such as meditation or merit seeking and actively participate in their treatment. The economy of hope surrounding assisted reproduction is both a moral economy and capital economy involving the circulation of values that are both ethical and commercial.

For many of the individual women and men with whom I spoke in the course of this study, initial enthusiasm and hope that assisted reproductive technologies would allow them to form a family gave way to dismay and disappointment. I documented some of their struggles and pragmatic choices to undergo treatment. Women are subjected to arduous, expensive, invasive and often agonizing interventions for IVF, in some cases iatrogenic interventions that further complicate their infertility. Throughout this book, pain is the background to many of the women's stories – the sheer visceral impact of surgeries to investigate the reproductive tract, clear, straighten and widen fallopian tubes, curettes to clean out the endometrium, let alone the daily injections into the abdomen, the surgery to 'harvest' eggs from ovaries and the loss of pregnancies. The pain is also existential as women question their inability to fulfil their desires to be a 'good' wife, mother and daughter-in-law, their futures, their relationships, the karmic misfortune of past lives. Women present themselves as proactive, making choices to deploy their bodies and use cutting-edge technologies in pursuit of their dream child. But this is not without contradictions; at the same time many women live within patriarchal bargains, they may give up their independence, their jobs and find themselves reduced to mere vessels as they become medicalized and enmeshed in the process.

Ultimately, behind any discussion of reproductive technologies lie questionable assumptions of the inevitable progress of science, the desirability of controlling reproduction and the perfectability of technology and the human being. As new assisted reproductive technologies are invented, societies will face further challenging ethical questions as to the desirability of limiting our experimentation with life. Ethnographies in different settings deny the universality of normative philosophical ethical claims; they demonstrate that local specificities and an understanding of actors' contexts and motives is required to debate different ethical positions. At stake in the stories presented in this book then is not just the production of embryos and families, not just the capacity of sexed bodies to reproduce, but the remaking of reproduction as a process and the questioning of how this should be done. It is through ethnographies that we can explore how differing societies grapple with our biofutures.

APPENDIX

Total Number of Interviewed Patients in Private and Public Clinics by Age, Sex and Education

		Age											
		Private Hospital				Subtotal	Public Hospital					Subtotal	Total
Sex	**Education**	**30–34**	**35–39**	**40–44**	**45–49**		**25–29**	**30–34**	**35–39**	**40–44**	**45–49**		
Female	**Primary school**							1				1	1
	Secondary school			1		1	2		1			3	4
	Undergrad	2	2	1		5	1		3	1		5	10
	Postgrad		1			1			1			1	2
	Unknown	2	2			4	1	3	2	3	1	10	14
Female Total		4	5	2		11	4	4	7	4	1	20	31
Male	**Primary school**									1		1	1
	Secondary school						1					1	1
	Undergrad	1				1			1			1	2
	Postgrad				1	1							1
	Unknown		3		2	5		1		2		3	8
Male Total		1	3		3	7	1	1	1	3		6	13
Total		5	8	2	3	18	5	5	8	7	1	26	44

Glossary

artificial insemination: Procedures involving the insertion of sperm within a woman's genital tract by a method other than sexual intercourse (see IUI).

donor eggs: Ova retrieved from one woman are given to an infertile woman for use in assisted reproductive procedures.

donor insemination: The use of the sperm of a man other than the recipient's partner for the purposes of achieving a pregnancy.

ectopic pregnancy: A condition in which a fertilized egg begins to develop in places other than within a woman's uterus (usually the fallopian tube, ovary or abdominal cavity). It causes pain and can cause rupture of a fallopian tube and potentially fatal internal bleeding.

embryo transfer: The procedure during which an embryo fertilized and developed in vitro is introduced into a woman's uterus.

endometrium: The lining of the uterus which is shed each month during menstruation and provides a site for implantation of fertilized eggs.

follicle: The cyst under the surface of the ovary in which an egg matures and is later released.

gestational surrogacy: Involves a woman who is not genetically related to the child who carries a pregnancy and delivers a baby for an infertile couple (cf. traditional surrogacy)

GIFT (gamete intrafallopian transfer): A technique in which a woman's ovum is removed from her ovaries and placed within one of her fallopian tubes directly with male sperm via laparoscopy. Fertilization takes place within the woman's uterus. This technique is used less often nowadays as IVF has similar success rates.

ICSI (intracytoplasmic sperm injection): Involves the micromanipulation of sperm to inject selected spermatozoa under the membrane surrounding an egg. Used in cases of male infertility.

IUI (intrauterine insemination): The technique of placing sperm directly into the uterine cavity. It is often one of the first and least expensive interventions attempted, especially in cases of cervical factors involved in infertility or unexplained cases of infertility. It may be used in combination with oral or injectable medications to stimulate ovulation.

implantation: Refers to the embedding of a fertilized egg into the endometrium.

IVF (in vitro fertilization): The process during which eggs are surgically removed from a woman's ovaries and combined outside the body with sperm in a laboratory dish. Following fertilization, the resultant fertilized eggs are left to develop for a number of days depending on the procedure before being returned to a woman's uterus or being frozen, discarded or donated.

oocyte, ovum: The female reproductive cell developed in the ovary or an egg.

oocyte retrieval: Also commonly known as oocyte harvesting. Involves a surgical procedure in which a needle is inserted into the ovarian follicles and the fluid and eggs are aspirated into the needle and then to a laboratory dish.

PGD (preimplantation genetic diagnosis): The screening and genetic diagnosis of a zygote or embryo while still developing in vitro by examining its chromosomes after the biopsy of a single cell. A controversial procedure that is banned in a number of countries, it can be used to screen for a range of genetic anomalies as well as sex-linked diseases or may be used to select for embryos of desired genetic characteristics as in the production of 'saviour siblings'. It may also be used for nonmedical purposes such as sex selection. Only embryos of the desired characteristics will be later transferred to a woman's uterus.

PID (pelvic inflammatory disease): Any form of inflammatory disease affecting the pelvis. Is an important cause of infertility due to scarring.

selective reduction: The reduction of one or more embryos in cases of multiple gestation. IVF technologies typically involve the production of multiple embryos. In the past, four embryos were typically transferred to a woman's uterus to maximize chances of a successful implantation and pregnancy. This practice increases the risk of higher-order multiple pregnancies. Because of the medical risks involved, patients carrying triplets or higher may be offered the option of a selective reduction in which a needle is inserted into the abdominal wall and potassium chloride is injected to stop the heart beating of one or more individual foetuses. This practice is highly controversial and rarely discussed in Thailand where abortion is highly stigmatized and highly restricted. Protocols in most clinics now discourage the transfer of multiple embryos, limiting it to two embryos to avoid higher-order multiple pregnancies and the need for selective reduction.

traditional surrogacy: In this form of surrogacy, a woman who is to carry the pregnancy uses her eggs in the procedures, either conceiving through insemination with the sperm of the partner of the infertile woman, sexual intercourse or through donor insemination. The resultant child is the genetic offspring of the surrogate.

variocele: A condition in men in which varicose veins form around the testicle.

ZIFT (zygote intrafallopian transfer): Following in vitro fertilization procedures, the early embryo (zygote) is placed in the fallopian tube via laparoscopy.

References

Adams, M. 2010. 'New Draft Law to Regulate Surrogacy in Thailand', 24 June 2010. *Thailand Law Forum: Law Analysis and Features on Southeast Asia.* http://www.thailawforum.com/new-draft-surrogacy-law-thailand.html (retrieved 1 May 2014).

Akande, E. O. 2008. 'Affordable Assisted Reproductive Technologies in Developing Countries: Pros and Cons', *Human Reproduction* 2008(1): 12–14.

Anatavuthikanon, S. 1992. 'Psychological Factors in Infertile Female [*sic*] at Infertility Clinic, Chulalongkorn Hospital'. MA dissertation. Bangkok: Chulalongkorn University (in Thai).

Alliance Anti Trafic (AAT). 2012. *Flash News: The Verdict of Thailand's First Forced Surrogacy Case Has Been Announced!* June 2012, no. 8. ftp://ftp2.allianceantitrafic.org/alliancea/2012%20Newsletters/flashnewsno.8.pdf (retrieved 21 May 2014).

Alliance Anti Trafic (AAT) Vietnam. 2011. *Follow-up Report on Surrogate Mothers' Case.* ftp://ftp2.allianceantitrafic.org/alliancea/000%20Surrogate%20mothers%20case%20in%20Vietnam%20and%20Thailand (retrieved 20 July 2013).

Appadurai, A. 1996. *Modernity at Large: Cultural Dimensions of Globalization.* Minneapolis: University of Minnesota Press.

Arditti, R., R. D. Klein and S. Minden (eds.). 1984. *Test-Tube Women: What Future Motherhood?* London: Pandora.

Askew, M. 2008. 'Materializing Merit: The Symbolic Economy of Religious Monuments and Tourist-Pilgrimage in Contemporary Thailand', in P. Kitiarsa (ed.), *Religious Commodifications in Asia.* London: Routledge, 89–119.

Becker, G. 2000. *The Elusive Embryo: How Women and Men Approach New Reproductive Technologies.* Berkeley: University of California Press.

Bennett, L. R. 2012. 'Infertility, Womanhood and Motherhood in Contemporary Indonesia: Understanding Gender Discrimination in the Realm of Biomedical Fertility Care', *Intersections: Gender and Sexuality in Asia and the Pacific* (28). http://intersections.anu.edu.au/issue28/bennett.htm (retrieved 1 May 2014).

Berkhout, S. G. 2008. 'Buns in the Oven: Objectification, Surrogacy, and Women's Autonomy', *Social Theory and Practice* 34(1): 95–117.

Bhagwati, J. 2002. 'Deconstructing Rotten Trade', *SAIS Review* 22(1): 39–44.

Bharadwaj, A. 2002. 'Conception Politics: Medical Egos, Media Spotlights, and the Contest over Test-Tube Firsts in India', in M. C Inhorn and F. van Balen (eds.), *Infertility Around the Globe: New Thinking on Childlessness, Gender, and Reproductive Technologies.* Berkeley: University of California Press, 315–333.

———. 2006a. 'Sacred Conceptions: Clinical Theodicies, Uncertain Science and Technologies of Procreation in India', *Culture, Medicine and Psychiatry* 30(4): 451–65.

———. 2006b. 'Sacred Modernity: Religion, Infertility and Technoscientific Conception around the Globe', *Culture, Medicine and Psychiatry* 30(4): 423–25.

———. 2008. 'Biosociality and Biocrossings: Encounters with Assisted Conception and Embryonic Stem Cells in India', in S. Gibbon and C. Novas (eds.), *Biosocialities, Genetics and the Social Sciences: Making Biologies and Identities.* Abingdon: Routledge, 98–116.

———. 2009. 'Assisted Life: The Neoliberal Moral Economy of Embryonic Stem Cells in India', in D. Birenbaum-Carmeli and M. C. Inhorn (eds.), *Assisting Reproduction, Testing Genes: Global Encounters with Technologies.* New York and Oxford: Berghahn Books, 239–57.

Birenbaum-Carmeli, D. 2007. 'Contested Surrogacy and the Gender Order: An Israeli Case Study', *Journal of Middle East Women's Studies* 3(3): 21–44.

Birenbaum-Carmeli, D., and M. C. Inhorn (eds.). 2009. *Assisting Reproduction, Testing Genes: Global Encounters with Technologies.* New York and Oxford: Berghahn Books.

Birke, L., S. Himmelweit and G. Vines. 1990. *Tomorrow's Child: Reproductive Technologies in the 90s.* London: Virago.

Boivin, J., et al. 2007. 'International Estimate of Infertility Prevalence and Treatment-Seeking: Potential Need and Demand for Infertility Medical Care', *Human Reproduction* 22(6): 1506–512.

Bonaccorso, M. M. E. 2009. *Conceiving Kinship: Assisted Conception, Procreation and Family in Southern Europe.* New York: Berghahn Books.

Boonmongkon, P. 1997. 'Living Through Infertility: From Loss to Resolution Over the Life Course of Thai Women', in V. Somswasdi and S. Theobald (eds.), *Women, Gender Relations and Development in Thai Society.* Chiang Mai: Women Studies Center, Faculty of Social Sciences, Chiang Mai University, 499–516.

Boris, E., and R. S. Parrenas. 2010. 'Introduction', in E. Boris and R. S. Parrenas (eds.), *Intimate Labors: Cultures, Technologies and the Politics of Care.* Stanford, CA: Stanford University Press, 1–12.

Bruckman, A. S. 1996. 'Gender Swapping on the Internet', in P. Ludlow (ed.), *High Noon on the Electric Frontier.* Cambridge, MA: MIT Press.

Carmeli, Y. S., and D. Birenbaum-Carmeli. 1994. 'The Predicament of Masculinity: Towards Understanding the Male's Experiences of Infertility Treatments', *Sex Roles* 30(9–10): 663–77.

Castells, M. 2000. *The Information Age: Economy, Society and Culture,* vol. 1. Oxford: Blackwell Publishers.

Chanrachakul, B., Y. Herabutya and U. Udomsubpayakul. 2000. 'Epidemic of Cesarean Section at the General, Private and University Hospitals in Thailand'. *Journal of Obstetrics and Gynecology Research* 26(5): 357–61.

Chaw-wattanakun, K. 2004. *The Socio-Cultural Construction of Stigma in Infertile Women.* MA dissertation. Bangkok: Chulalongkorn University (in Thai).

Chiamchanya, C., and W. Su-angkawatin. 2008. 'Study of the Causes and the Results of Treatment in Infertile Couples at Thammasat Hospital between 1999–2004', *Journal of the Medical Association of Thailand = Chotmaihet Thangphaet* 91(6): 805–12.

Choavaratana, R., S. Suppinyopong and P. Chaimahaphruksa. 1999. 'ROSI from TESE the First Case in Thailand: A Case Report', *Journal of the Medical Association of Thailand = Chotmaihet Thangphaet* 82(9): 938–41.

Cohen, E. 1992. 'Pilgrimage Centers: Concentric and Eccentric', *Annals of Tourism Research* 19(1): 33–50.

Corea, G. 1988. *The Mother Machine: Reproductive Technologies from Artificial Insemination to Artificical Wombs.* London: Women's Press.

Corea, G., et al. 1987. *Man-Made Women: How New Reproductive Technologies Affect Women.* Bloomington: Indiana University Press.

Das, V. 2001. 'Stigma, Contagion, Defect: Issues in the Anthropology of Public Health', *Stigma and Global Health Conference,* 5–7 September 2001. Bethesda, MD: National Institutes of Health.

Davis, A. 1998. 'Surrogates and Outcast Mothers: Racism and Reproductive Politics in the Nineties', in J. James (ed.), *The Angela Y. Davis Reader.* Oxford: Blackwell, 210–21.

De Rosa, M., et al. 2003. 'Traffic Pollutants Affect Fertility in Men', *Human Reproduction* 18(5): 1055–61.

DeLanda, M. 2002. *Intensive Science and Virtual Philosophy.* London: Continuum.

Deleuze, G., and F. Guattari. 2003. *A Thousand Plateaus.* Minneapolis: University of Minnesota Press.

Dissanayake V. H. W, R. Simpson and R. W. Jayasekara. 2002. 'Attitudes Towards the New Genetic and Assisted Reproductive Technologies in Sri Lanka: A Preliminary Report', *New Genetics and Society* 21(1): 65–74.

Donchin, A. 2010. 'Reproductive Tourism and the Quest for Global Gender Justice', *Bioethics* 24(7): 323–32.

Dworkin, A. 1983. *Right-Wing Women.* New York: Perigee Books.

Farquhar, J. 1991. 'Objects, Processes and Female Infertility in Chinese Medicine', *Medical Anthropology Quarterly* 5(4): 370–99.

Ford, N., and S. Kittisuksathit. 1994. 'Destinations Unknown: The Gender Construction and Changing Nature of the Sexual Lifestyles of Thai Youth', *AIDS Care* 6(5): 517–31.

Ford, N., et al. 2004. 'The Role of Civil Society in Protecting Public Health over Commercial Interests: Lessons from Thailand', *The Lancet* 363(9408): 560–63.

Ford, N., et al. 2009. 'Challenge and Co-Operation: Civil Society Activism for Access to HIV Treatment in Thailand', *Tropical Medicine and International Health* 14(3): 258–66.

Fordham, G. 2004. *A New Look At Thai Aids: Perspectives from The Margin.* Oxford and New York: Berghahn Books.

Foucault, M. 1984. *The History of Sexuality.* London: Penguin.

Foucault, M., and G. Deleuze. 1977. 'Intellectuals and Power', in D. F. Bouchard (ed.), *Language, Counter-Memory, Practice: Selected Essays and Interviews.* Ithaca, NY: Cornell University Press, 205–17.

Franklin, S. 1990. 'Deconstructing "Desperateness": The Social Construction of Infertility in Popular Representations of New Reproductive Technologies', in M. McNeil, J. Varcoe and S. Yearley (eds.), *The New Reproductive Technologies.* New York: St. Martin's Press, 220–29.

———. 1997. *Embodied Progress: A Cultural Account of Assisted Conception.* London and New York: Routledge.

———. 1998. 'Making Miracles: Scientific Progress and the Facts of Life', in S. Franklin and H. Ragone (eds.), *Reproducing Reproduction: Kinship, Power and Reproduction.* Philadelphia: University of Pennsylvania Press, 102–17.

Garcia, A. C., et al. 2009. 'Ethnographic Approaches to the Internet and Computer-Mediated Communication', *Journal of Contemporary Ethnography* 38(1): 52–84.

Gell, A. 1992. 'The Technology of Enchantment and the Enchantment of Technology', in J. Coote and A. Shelton (eds.), *Anthropology, Art and Aesthetics.* Oxford: Clarendon, 40–66.

———. 1993. *Wrapping in Images: Tattooing in Polynesia.* Oxford: Clarendon Press.

Gerrits, T. 2002. 'Infertility and Matrilineality: The Exceptional Case of the Macua of Mozambique', in M. Inhorn and F. van Balen (eds.), *Infertility around the Globe: New Thinking on Childlessness, Gender and Reproductive Technologies.* Berkeley: University of California Press, 233–46.

Gesler, W. M. 1996. 'Lourdes: Healing in a Place of Pilgrimage', *Health and Place* 2(2): 95–105.

Ginsburg, F., and R. Rapp. 1991. 'The Politics of Reproduction', *Annual Review of Anthropology* 20: 311–43.

Golomb, L. 1985. *An Anthropology of Curing in Multiethnic Thailand.* Chicago: University of Illinois Press.

———. 2000. 'Body Boundaries, Fiction of the Female Self: An Ethnographic Perspective on Power, Feminism, and the Reproductive Technologies', *Feminist Studies* 26(1): 113–40.

Greil, A. L., T. A. Leitko and K. L. Porter. 1988. 'Infertility: His and Hers', *Gender and Society* 2(2): 172–99.

Gurunath, S., et al. 2011. 'Defining Infertility: A Systematic Review of Prevalence Studies', *Human Reproduction Update* 17(5): 575–88.

Haggerty, K. D., and R. V. Ericson. 2000. 'The Surveillant Assemblage', *The British Journal of Sociology* 51(4): 605–22.

Handwerker, L. 2002. 'The Politics of Making Modern Babies in China: Reproductive Technologies and the "New" Eugenics', in M. C. Inhorn and F. van Balen (eds.), *Infertility around the Globe: New Thinking on Childlessness, Gender and Reproductive Technologies.* Berkeley: University of California Press, 298–314.

Haora, P. J. 2013. 'From Home to Hospital: "Safe Motherhood", Hospitalisation and the Birthing Transition in Thailand (1945–2006)'. PhD dissertation. Canberra: Australian National University.

Haraway, D. 1991. *Simians, Cyborgs and Women: The Reinvention of Nature.* New York: Chapman and Hall.

Harding, S. G. 1991. *Whose Science? Whose Knowledge? Thinking from Women's Lives.* Ithaca, NY: Cornell University Press.

Healy, D. L., A. O. Trounson and A. N. Andersen. 1994. 'Female Infertility: Causes and Treatment', *The Lancet* 343(8912): 1539–544.

Heath, D., R. Rapp and K.-S. Taussig. 2004. 'Genetic Citizenship', in D. Nugent and J. Vincent (eds.), *A Companion to the Anthropology of Politics.* London: Blackwell, 152–67.

Heinze, R. I. 1988. *Trance and Healing in Southeast Asia Today.* Bangkok: White Lotus.

Inhorn, M. C. 1994. *Quest for Conception: Gender, Infertility and Eygptian Medical Traditions.* Philadelphia: University of Pennsylvania Press.

———. 1996. *Infertility and Patriarchy: The Cultural Politics of Gender and Family Life in Egypt.* Philadelphia: University of Pennslyvania Press.

———. 2000. 'Missing Motherhood: Infertility, Technology and Poverty in Egyptian Women's Lives', in H. Ragone and F. W. Twine (eds.), *Ideologies and Technologies of Motherhood: Race, Class, Sexuality, Nationalism.* New York: Routledge, 139–68.

———. 2002. 'Sexuality, Masculinity, and Infertility in Egypt: Potent Troubles in the Marital and Medical Encounters', *Journal of Men's Studies* 10(3): 343–59.

———. 2003a. *Local Babies, Global Science: Gender, Religion and in-Vitro Fertilization in Egypt.* New York: Routledge.

———. 2003b. 'Global Infertility and the Globalization of New Reproductive Technologies: Illustrations from Egypt', *Social Science and Medicine* 56(9): 1837–851.

———. 2004a. 'Privacy, Privatization, and the Politics of Patronage: Ethnographic Challenges to Penetrating the Secret World of Middle Eastern, Hospital-Based in Vitro Fertilization', *Social Science and Medicine* 59(10): 2095–108.

———. 2004b. 'Middle Eastern Masculinities in the Age of New Reproductive Technologies: Male Infertility and Stigma in Egypt and Lebanon', *Medical Anthropology Quarterly* 18(2): 162–82.

———. 2006a. '"He Won't Be My Son": Middle Eastern Muslim Men's Discourses of Adoption and Gamete Donation', *Medical Anthropology Quarterly* 20(1): 94–120.

———. 2006b. 'Making Muslim Babies: IVF and Gamete Donation in Sunni Versus Shi'a Islam', *Culture, Medicine and Psychiatry* 30(4): 427–50.

———. 2007a. 'Masculinity, Reproduction, and Male Infertility Surgery in the Middle East', *Journal of Middle East Women's Studies* 3(3): 1–20.

———. 2007b. 'Masturbation, Semen Collection and Men's IVF Experiences: Anxieties in the Muslim World', *Body and Society* 13(3): 37–53.

———. 2009. 'Right to Assisted Reproductive Technology: Overcoming Infertility in Low-Resource Countries', *International Journal of Gynaecology and Obstetrics* 106(2): 172–74.

———. 2011. 'Globalization and Gametes: Reproductive "Tourism", Islamic Bioethics, and Middle Eastern Modernity', *Anthropology and Medicine* 18(1): 87–103.

Inhorn, M. C., and E. A. Wentzell. 2011. 'Embodying Emergent Masculinities: Men Engaging with Reproductive and Sexual Health Technologies in the Middle East and Mexico', *American Ethnologist* 38(4): 801–15.

Inhorn, M. C., and D. Birenbaum-Carmeli. 2008. 'Assisted Reproductive Technologies and Culture Change', *Annual Review of Anthropology* 37: 177–96.

Irvine, W. 1982. 'The Thai- Yuan "Madman" and the "Modernising, Developing Thai Nation" as Bounded Entities under Threat: A Study in the Replication of a Single Image'. PhD dissertation. London: University of London.

Isidori, A., M. Latini and F. Romanelli. 2005. 'Treatment of Male Infertility', *Contraception* 72(4): 314–18.

Jackson, P. A. 1999a. 'The Enchanting Spirit of Thai Capitalism: The Cult of Luang Phor Khoon and the Post-Modernization of Thai Buddhism', *South East Asia Research* 7(1): 5–60.

———. 1999b. 'Royal Spirits, Chinese Gods and Magic Monks: Thailand's Boom Time Religions of Prosperity', *South East Asia Research* 7(3): 245–320.

———. 2000. 'An Explosion of Thai Identities: Global Queering and Re-Imagining Queer Theory', *Culture, Health and Sexuality* 2(4): 405–24.

Jackson, P. A., and N. M. Cook (eds.). 1999. *Genders and Sexualities in Modern Thailand.* Chiang Mai: Silkworm Books.

Jacobson, J. L. 2000. 'Transforming Family Planning Programmes: A Framework for Advancing the Reproductive Rights Agenda', *Reproductive Health Matters* 8(15): 21–32.

Jansen, W., and M. Kühl. 2008. 'Shared Symbols: Muslims, Marian Pilgrimages and Gender', *European Journal of Women's Studies* 15(3): 295–311.

Jensen, T. K., J. P. Bonde and M. Joffe. 2006. 'The Influence of Occupational Exposure on Male Reproductive Function', *Occupational Medicine* 56(8): 544–53.

Kahn, S. M. 2000. *Reproducing Jews: A Cultural Account of Assisted Conception in Israel.* Durham, NC: Duke University Press.

———. 2006. 'Making Technology Familiar: Orthodox Jews and Infertility Support, Advice, and Inspiration', *Culture, Medicine and Psychiatry* 30(4): 467–80.

Kandiyoti, D. 1991. 'Bargaining with Patriarchy', in J. Lorber and S. A. Farrell (eds.), *The Social Construction of Gender.* Newbury Park, CA: Sage Publications, 104–18

Kapferer, B. 2000. 'Star Wars: About Anthropology, Culture and Globalisation', *The Australian Journal of Anthropology* 11(2): 174–98.

Kato, M., and M. Sleeboom-Faulkner. 2011. 'Meanings of the Embryo in Japan: Narratives of IVF Experience and Embryo Ownership', *Sociology of Health and Illness* 33(3): 434–47.

Keown, D. 1995. *Buddhism and Bioethics.* London: Palgrave.

Keyes, C. F. 1984. 'Mother or Mistress but Never a Monk: Buddhist Notions of Female Gender in Rural Thailand', *American Ethnologist* 11(2): 223–41.

———. 2002. 'National Heroine or Local Spirit? The Struggle over Memory in the Case of Thao Suranari of Nakhon Ratchasimathe Struggle over Memory in the Case of Thao Suranari of Nakhon Ratchasima', in S. Tanabe and C. F. Keyes (eds.), *Cultural Crisis and Social Memory: Modernity and Identity in Thailand and Laos.* London: Routledge Curzon, 113–36.

———. 2006. 'The Destruction of a Shrine to Brahma in Bangkok and Fall of Thaksin Shinawatra: The Occult and the Thai Coup in Thailand of September 2006', *Asia Research Institute, Working Paper Series No. 80.* National University of Singapore.

Kirsch, A.T. 1982. 'Buddhism, Sex-Roles and the Thai Economy', in P. V. Esterik (ed.), *Women of Southeast Asia.* Detroit: Northern Illinois University, 16–41.

———. 1985. 'Text and Context: Buddhist Sex Roles – Culture of Gender Revisited', *American Ethnologist* 12(1): 302–20.

Kitiarsa, P. 2005. 'Beyond Syncretism: Hybridization of Popular Religion in Contemporary Thailand', *Journal of Southeast Asian Studies* 36(3): 461–87.

——— (ed.). 2007. *Religious Commodifications in Asia: Marketing Gods.* New York: Routledge.

Klausner, W. J. 1993. *Reflections on Thai Culture (Collected Writings).* Bangkok: The Siam Society.

Klein, R. 2008. 'From Test-Tube Women to Bodies without Women', *Women's Studies International Forum* 31: 157–75.

Knodel, J., et al. 1999. 'Sexuality, Sexual Experience, and the Good Spouse: Views of Married Thai Men and Women', in P. A. Jackson and N. M. Cook (eds.), *Genders and Sexualities in Modern Thailand.* Chiang Mai: Silkworm Books, 93–113.

Knodel, J., A. Chamratrithirong and N. Debavalya. 1987. *Thailand's Reproductive Revolution: Rapid Fertility Decline in a Third World Setting.* Madison: University of Wisconsin Press.

Konrad, M. 1998. 'Ova Donation and Symbols of Substance: Some Variations on the Theme of Sex, Gender and the Partible Body', *Journal of the Royal Anthropological Institute* 4(4): 643–67.

Krannich, R. L., and C. R. Krannich. 1980. *The Politics of Family Planning Policy: Thailand – A Case of Successful Implementation.* Berkeley: University of California, Center for South and Southeast Asia Studies Monograph Series No. 19.

Latour, B. 1993. *We Have Never Been Modern.* Cambridge, MA: Harvard University Press

Liamputtong, P. 2000. '"A Barren Body": The Cultural Interpretation of Infertility among Hmong Women in Australia', in F. van Balen, T. Gerrits and M. C. Inhorn (eds.), *Social Science Research on Childlessness in a Global Perspective: Proceedings of the Conference, 8–11 November 1999, Amsterdam, the Netherlands.* Amsterdam: SCO-Kohnstamm Instituut, University of Amsterdam.

———. 2009. 'Treating the Afflicted Body: Perceptions of Infertility and Ethnomedicine among Fertile Hmong Women in Australia', in F. Van Rooij, N. Hudson and L. Culley (eds.), *Marginalised Reproduction: Ethnicity, Infertility and Reproductive Technologies.* London: Earthscan.

Lloyd, M. 1996. 'Condemned to Be Meaningful: Non-Reponse in Studies of Men and Infertility', *Sociology of Health and Illness* 18(4): 433–54.

Lock, M. 1998. 'Perfecting Society: Reproductive Technologies, Genetic Testing, and the Planned Family in Japan', in M. Lock and P. A. Kaufert (eds.), *Pragmatic Women and Body Politics.* Cambridge: Cambridge University Press, 206–39.

Lock, M., and P. A. Kaufert. 1998. 'Introduction', in M. Lock and P. A. Kaufert (eds.), *Pragmatic Women and Body Politics.* Cambridge: Cambridge University Press, 1–27.

Loos, T. L. 1999. 'Gender Adjudicated: Translating Modern Legal Subjects in Siam'. PhD dissertation. Ithaca, NY: Cornell University.

Lorber, J. 1989. 'Choice, Gift or Patriarchal Bargain? Women's Conset to in Vitro Fertilization in Male Infertility', *Hypatia* 4: 23–36.

Lowry, D. W. 2004. 'Understanding Reproductive Technologies as a Surveillant Assemblage: Revisions of Power and Technoscience', *Sociological Perspectives* 47(4): 357–70.

Lyttleton, C., A. Beesey and M. Sitthikriengkrai. 2007. 'Expanding Community through ARV Provision in Thailand', *AIDS Care* 19(Suppl 1): S44–53.

Mahidol Population Gazette. 2007. Vol. 16. Salaya: Institute for Population and Social Research, Mahidol University.

Majupuria, T. C. 1987. *Erawan Shrine and Brahma Worship in Thailand with Reference to Nepal and India.* Bangkok: Craftsman Press.

Marcus, G. E., and E. Saka. 2006. 'Assemblage', *Theory, Culture, Society* 23(2–3): 101–6.

McGilvray, D. B. 1994. 'Sexual Power and Fertility in Sri Lanka: Batticaloa Tamils and Moors', in C. P. Maccormack (ed.), *Ethnography of Fertility and Birth,* 2nd ed. Prospect Heights, IL: Waveland Press Inc, 15–63.

McLelland, M. 2007. 'Internet Domains between China and India: Beyond Anglophone Paradigms', *Asian Studies Review* 31(4): 387–95.

Morris, R. C. 2000. *In the Place of Origins: Modernity and its Mediums in Northern Thailand.* Durham, NC: Duke University Press.

Muecke, M. A. 1984. 'Make Money Not Babies. Changing Status Markers of Northern Thai Women', *Anthropology Today* 26(4): 459–70.

———. 1992. 'Mother Sold Food, Daughter Sells Her Body: The Cultural Continuity of Prostitution', *Social Science and Medicine* 35(7): 891–901.

Mulholland, J. 1989. *Herbal Medicine in Paediatrics Translation of a Thai Book of Genesis.* Canberra: Faculty of Asian Studies, Australian National University.

Nachtigall, R. D., et al. 2005. '"Parents" Conceptualization of Their Frozen Embryos Complicates the Disposition Decision', *Fertility and Sterility* 84(2): 431–34.

Nahar, P. 2007. *Childless in Bangladesh: Suffering and Resilience among Rural and Urban Women.* Amsterdam: University of Amsterdam.

Nahar, P., et al. 2000. 'Living with Infertility: Experiences among Urban Slum Populations in Bangladesh', *Reproductive Health Matters* 8(15): 33–44.

Nahman, M. 2006. 'Materialising Israeliness: Difference and Mixture in Transnational Ova Donation', *Science as Culture* 15(3): 199–213.

———. 2011. 'Reverse Traffic: Intersecting Inequalities in Human Egg Donation', *Reproductive Biomedicine Online* 23(5): 626–33.

Neff, D. L. 1994. 'The Social Construction of Infertility: The Case of the Matrilineal Nayars in South India', *Social Science and Medicine* 39(4): 475–85.

Nilsen, M. 2011. 'The Spirit of a Heroine: Ya Mo – Spirit Reverence, Patriotism and Thai Buddhism', *Modern Asian Studies* 45(6): 1599–625.

Nortemans, C. 2007. 'Loss and Healing: A Marian Pilgrimage in Secular Dutch Society', *Ethnology* 46(3): 217–33.

O'Connor, R. A. 1993. 'Temples, Sangha Reform and Social Change', *Journal of Southeast Asian Studies* 24(2): 330–39.

Ombelet, W., et al. 2008. 'Infertility and the Provision of Infertility Medical Services in Developing Countries', *Human Reproduction* 14(6): 605–21.

Ong, A., and N. N. Chen (eds.). 2010. *Asian Biotech: Ethics and Communities of Fate.* Durham, NC: Duke University Press.

Ong, A., and S. Collier (eds.). 2005. *Global Assemblages: Technology, Politics, and Ethics as Anthropological Problems.* Oxford: Blackwell.

Packard-Winkler, M. 1996. 'Constructions of Knowledge and Discourse in Middle Class Marriage: Implications for Coping with Sexual Risk among Urban Thai'. 6th International Conference on Thai Studies, 14–17 October 1996. Chiang Mai, Thailand.

Padmavati, R., R. Thara and E. Corin. 2005. 'A Qualitative Study of Religious Practices by Chronic Mentally Ill and Their Caregivers in South India', *International Journal of Social Psychiatry* 51(2): 139–49.

Pande, A. 2009. 'Not an "Angel", not a "Whore": Surrogates as "Dirty" Workers in India', *Indian Journal of Gender Studies* 16(2): 141–73.

———. 2010. 'Commercial Surrogacy in India: Manufacturing a Perfect Mother-Worker', *Signs: Journal of Women in Culture and Society* 35(4): 969–94.

———. 2011. 'Transnational Commercial Surrogacy in India: Gifts for Global Sisters?', *Reproductive Biomedicine Online* 23(5): 618–25.

Parks, J. 2010. 'Care Ethics and the Global Practice of Commercial Surrogacy', *Bioethics* 24(7): 333–40.

Pashigan, M. J. 2002. 'Conceiving the Happy Family: Infertility and Marital Politics in Northern Vietnam', in M. Inhorn and F. van Balen (eds.), *Infertility Around the Globe: New Thinking on Childlessness, Gender and Reproductive Technologies.* Berkeley: University of California Press, 134–51.

———. 2009. 'The Womb, Infertility and the Vicissitudes of Kin-Relatedness in Vietnam', *Journal of Vietnamese Studies* 4(2): 34–68.

Paxson, H. 2003. 'With or Against Nature? IVF, Gender and Reproductive Agency in Athens, Greece', *Social Science and Medicine* 56(9): 1853–866.

———. 2006. 'Reproduction as Spiritual Kin Work: Orthodoxy, IVF, and the Moral Economy of Motherhood in Greece', *Culture, Medicine and Psychiatry* 30(4): 481–505.

Pfeffer, N. 1993. *The Stork and the Syringe: A Political History of Reproductive Medicine.* Cambridge: Polity Press.

Pfleiderer, B. 1988. 'The Semiotics of Ritual Healing in a North Indian Musim Shrine', *Social Science and Medicine* 27(5): 417–24.

Pickering, A. 1992. 'From Science as Knowledge to Science as Practice', in A. Pickering (ed.), *Science as Practice and Culture.* Chicago, IL: University of Chicago Press, 1–26.

Pirani, F., et al. 2008. '"I Will Accept Whatever Is Meant for Us. I Will Wait for That – Day and Night": The Search for Healing at a Muslim Shrine in Pakistan', *Mental Health, Religion and Culture* 11(4): 375–86.

Practice Committee of the American Society for Reproductive Medicine. 2012. 'Multiple Gestation Associated with Infertility Therapy: An American Society for Reproductive Medicine Practice Committee Opinion', *Fertility and Sterility* 97(4): 825–34.

Rabinow, P. 1996. 'Artificiality and Enligtenment: From Sociobiology to Biosociality', in P. Rabinow (ed.), *Essays on the Anthropology of Reason.* Princeton, NJ: Princeton University Press, 91–111.

———. 2003. *Anthropos Today.* Princeton, NJ: Princeton University Press.

Ragoné, H., and F. W. Twine (eds.). 2000. *Ideologies and Technologies of Motherhood: Race, Class, Sexuality, Nationalism.* New York: Routledge.

Ragoné, H. 1994. *Surrogate Motherhood: Conception in the Heart.* Boulder, CO: Westview Press.

———. 2000. 'Of Likeness and Difference: How Race Is Being Transfigured by Gestational Surrogacy', in H. Ragoné and F. W. Twine (eds.), *Ideologies and Technologies of Motherhood: Race, Class, Sexuality, Nationalism.* New York: Routledge, 1–7.

———. 2005. 'Surrogate Motherhood: Rethinking Biological Models, Kinship, and Family', in C. B. Brettell and C. F. Sargent (eds.), *Gender in Cross-Cultural Perspective.* Upper Saddle River, NJ: Prentice Hall, 471–80.

Raguram, R., et al. 2002. 'Traditional Community Resources for Mental Health: A Report of Temple Healing from India', *British Medical Journal* 325(7354): 38–40.

Rapp, R. 1987. 'Moral Pioneers: Women, Men and Foetuses on a Frontier of Reproductive Technology', *Women and Health* 13(1–2): 101–16.

———. 1990. 'Constructing Amniocentesis: Maternal and Medical Discourse', in F. Ginsburg and A. L. Tsing (eds.), *Uncertain Terms: Negotiating Gender in American Culture*. Boston, MA: Beacon Press, 28–42.

———. 1999. *Testing Women, Testing the Fetus: The Social Impact of Amniocentesis in America*. New York: Routledge.

Raspberry, K. 2009. 'The Genesis of Embryos and Ethics in Vitro: Practicing Preimplantation Genetic Diagnosis in Argentina', in D. Birenbaum-Carmeli and M. C. Inhorn (eds.), *Assisting Reproduction, Testing Genes: Global Encounters with Technologies*. New York and Oxford: Berghahn Books, 213–38.

Rashid, S. F. 2007. 'Durbolota (Weakness), Chinta Rog (Worry Illness), and Poverty: Explanations of White Discharge among Married Adolescent Women in an Urban Slum in Dhaka, Bangladesh', *Medical Anthropology Quarterly* 21(1): 108–32.

Ratanakul, P. 1999. 'Socio-Medical Aspects of Abortion in Thailand', in D. Keown (ed.), *Buddhism and Abortion*. Honolulu: University of Hawai'i Press, 53–66.

Raymond, J. G. 1995. *Women as Wombs: Reproductive Technologies and the Battle over Women's Freedom*. North Melbourne: Spinifex Press.

Rheingold, H. 1993. *The Virtual Community: Homesteading on the Electronic Frontier*. Reading, MI: Addison-Wesley Publishing Company.

Riessman, C. K. 2000. 'Stigma and Everyday Resistance Practices: Childless Women in South India', *Gender and Society* 14(1): 111–35.

———. 2002. 'Positioning Gender Identity in Narratives of Infertility: South Indian Women's Lives in Context', in M. C. Inhorn and F. van Balen (eds.), *Infertility Around the Globe: New Thinking on Childlessness, Gender and Reproductive Technologies*. Berkeley: University of California Press, 152–70.

Roberts, D. 1995. 'Race and the New Reproduction', *Hastings Law Journal* 47(4): 935–49.

Roberts, E. F. S. 1998. 'Examining Surrogacy Discourses between Feminine Power and Exploitation', in N. Scheper-Hughes and C. Sargent (eds.), *Small Wars: The Cultural Politics of Childhood*. Berkley, Los Angeles and London: University of California Press, 93–110.

———. 2006. 'God's Laboratory: Religious Rationalities and Modernity in Ecuadorian in Vitro Fertilization', *Culture, Medicine and Psychiatry* 30(4): 507–36.

———. 2008. 'Biology, Sociality and Reproductive Modernity in Ecuadorian *in-Vitro* Fertilization: The Particulars of Place', in S. Gibbon and C. Novas (eds.), *Biosocialities, Genetics and the Social Sciences: Making Biologies and Identities*. Abingdon, VA: Routledge, 79–97.

———. 2009. 'The Traffic Between Women: Female Alliance and Familial Egg Donation in Ecuador', in D. Birenbaum-Carmeli and M. C. Inhorn (eds.), *Assisting Reproduction, Testing Genes: Global Encounters with Technologies.* New York and Oxford: Berghahn Books, 113–43.

Rose, N. 2007. *The Politics of Life Itself: Biomedicine, Power and Subjectivity in the Twenty-First Century.* Princeton, NJ: Princeton University Press.

Rose, N., and C. Novas. 2005. 'Biological Citizenship', in A. Ong and S. J. Collier (eds.), *Global Assemblages: Technology, Politics and Ethics as Anthropological Problems.* Malden, MA: Blackwell Publishing, 439–63.

Rothman, B. K. 1988. 'Reproductive Technology and the Commodification of Life', in E. Hoffman Baruch, A. F. D'Adamo Jr. and J. Seager (eds.), *Embryos, Ethics, and Women's Rights: Exploring the New Reproductive Technologies.* New York: Haworth, 95–100.

———. 1989. *Recreating Motherhood: Ideology and Technology in a Patriarchal Society.* New York: Norton.

Royal Thai Government Gazette. 2005. Thai Medical Council's Regulation on Criteria for Performing Therapeutic Termination of Pregnancy in Accordance with Section 305 of the Criminal Code, vol. 122, section 118 Ngor, 7–8.

Saengtienchai, C., et al. 1999. '"Prostitutes Are Better Than Lovers": Wives' Views on the Extramarital Sexual Behaviour of Thai Men', in P. A. Jackson and N. M. Cook (eds.), *Genders and Sexualities in Modern Thailand.* Chiang Mai: Silkworm Books, 78–92.

Sandelowski, M. 1990. 'Fault Lines: Infertility and Imperiled Sisterhood', *Feminist Studies* 16(1): 33–52.

———. 1991. 'Compelled to Try: The Never-Enough Quality of Conceptive Technology', *Medical Anthropology Quarterly* 5(1): 29–47.

———. 1993. *With Child in Mind: Studies of the Personal Encounter with Infertility.* Philadelphia: University of Pennsylvania Press.

Sandelowski, M., and S. de Lacey. 2002. 'The Uses of a "Disease": Infertility as Rhetorical Vehicle', in M. C. Inhorn and F. van Balen (eds.), *Infertility Around the Globe: New Thinking on Childlessness, Gender, and Reproductive Technologies.* Berkeley: University of California Press, 33–51.

Simpson, B., V. H. W. Dissanayake and R. W. Jayasekara. 2005. 'Contemplating Choice: Attitudes Towards Intervening in Human Reproduction in Sri Lanka', *New Genetics And Society* 24(1): 99–117.

Sparkes, S. 1995. 'Taming Nature – Controlling Fertility: Concepts of Nature and Gender among the Isan of Northeast Thailand', in O. Bruun and A. Kalland (eds.), *Asian Perceptions of Nature: A Critical Approach.* Surrey: Curzon Press, 63–87.

Sreeyamart, P. 2004. 'Perception and Coping Behavior among Infertile Couples'. MA dissertation. Thailand: Khon Kaen University.

Srivichai, S. 2001. 'Powerlessness of Women with Infertility'. MA dissertation. Thailand: Chiang Mai University.

Stanworth, M. (ed.). 1987. *Reproductive Technologies: Gender, Motherhood, and Medicine.* Cambridge. Oxford: Polity Press, in association with B. Blackwell.

Strathern, M. 1992. *Reproducing the Future: Anthropology, Kinship and the New Reproductive Technologies.* New York: Routledge.

Stott, P. 1991. 'Mu'ang and Pa: Elite Views of Nature in a Changing Thailand', in M. Chitakasem and A. Turton (eds.), *Thai Constructions of Knowledge.* London: School of Oriental and African Studies, 142–54.

Tangcharoensathien, V., et al. 2002. 'Caesarean Deliveries in Thailand: Cause for Concern', *Regional Health Forum* (online), 6. http://www.webcitation.org/5hSlQK5gE (retrieved 20 August 2013).

Taylor, J. 2008. *Buddhism and Postmodern Imaginings in Thailand: The Religiosity of Urban Space.* Farnham: Ashgate.

Teerapong, S. 2001. คนมีลูกยาก คนอยากมีลูก *Khon Mii Luuk Yaak Khon Yak Mii Luuk* (Those Who Have Difficulties Having a Baby / Those Who Want to Have a Baby). Bangkok: Sukaphapjai.

Teman, E. 2001. 'Technological Fragmentation and Women's Empowerment: Surrogate Motherhood in Israel', *Women's Studies Quarterly* 29(3–4): 11–34.

———. 2003. 'The Medicalization of "Nature" in the "Artificial Body": Surrogate Motherhood in Israel', *Medical Anthropology Quarterly* 17(1): 78–98.

———. 2010. *Birthing a Mother: The Surrogate Body and the Pregnant Self.* Berkeley: University of California Press.

Thompson, C. 2002. 'Fertile Ground: Feminists Theorize Infertility', in M. Inhorn and F. van Balen (eds.), *Infertility Around the Globe: New Thinking on Childlessness, Gender and Reproductive Technologies.* Berkeley: University of California Press, 52–78.

———. 2005. *Making Parents: The Ontological Choreography of Reproductive Technologies.* Cambridge, MA: MIT Press.

Threechana and C. Pimonsing. 2004. อยากเป็นแม่แค่ขาดใจ Yaak *pen mae khae khaadjai (I Want to Be a Mother Until I Die): Mommy's Story.* Bangkok: Kantana Publishing.

Tremayne, S. 2006. 'Not All Muslims Are Luddites', *Anthropology Today* 22(3): 1–2.

———. 2009. 'Law, Ethics and Donor Technologies in Shia Iran', in D. Birenbaum-Carmeli and M. C. Inhorn (eds.), *Assisting Reproduction, Testing Genes: Global Encounters with Technologies.* New York and Oxford: Berghahn Books, 144–63.

Turner, V., and E. Turner. 1978. *Image and Pilgrimage in Christian Culture.* Oxford: Basil Blackwell.

United Nations Population Fund (UNFPA). 2005. 'Reproductive Health of Women in Thailand: Progress and Challenge Towards Attainment of International Development Goals'. Bangkok.

Unnithan-Kumar, M. 2003. 'Spirits of the Womb: Migration, Reproductive Choice and Healing in Rajasthan', *Contributions to Indian Sociology* 37(1–2): 163–88.

van Balen, F. 2009. 'Infertility and Culture: Explanations, Implications and Dilemmas', in F. Van Rooij, N. Hudson and L. Culley (eds.), *Marginal-*

ized Reproduction: Ethnicity, Infertility and Reproductive Technologies. London: Earthscan, 33–48.
van Balen, F., and M. C. Inhorn. 2002. 'Introduction. Interpreting Infertility: A View from the Social Sciences', in M. C. Inhorn and F. van Balen (eds.), *Infertility Around the Globe: New Thinking on Childlessness, Gender, and Reproductive Technologies.* Berkeley: University of California Press, 3–32.
Van Esterik, P. 2000. *Materializing Thailand.* Oxford: Berg.
van Gennep, A. 1960. *The Rites of Passage.* London: Routledge and Kegan Paul.
van Niekerk, A., and L. van Zyl. 1995. 'The Ethics of Surrogacy: Women's Reproductive Labour', *Journal of Medical Ethics* 21(6): 345–49.
Vayena, E., et al. 2009. 'Assisted Reproductive Technologies in Developing Countries: Are We Caring Yet?', *Fertility and Sterility* 92(2): 413–16.
Virutamasen, P., et al. 2001. 'The Regulation of Assisted Reproductive Technology in Thailand', *Journal of the Medical Association of Thailand* 84(10): 1490–494.
Vora, K. 2010. 'Medicine, Markets and the Pregnant Body: Indian Commercial Surrogacy and Reproductive Labor in a Transnational Frame', *S&F Online (The Scholar and Feminist Online)* 9(1–2). http://sfonline.barnard.edu/reprotech/vora_01.htm (retrieved 6 May 2014).
Vutyavanich, T., et al. 2011. 'Assisted Reproductive Technologies in Thailand: 2001–2007 Results Generated from the Art Registry, Royal Thai College of Obstetricians and Gynaecologists', *Journal Of Obstetrics And Gynaecology Research* 37(3): 236–44.
Walsh, M. 2007. 'Efficacious Surroundings: Temple Space and Buddhist Well-Being', *Journal of Religion and Health* 46(4): 471–79.
Whittaker, A. 1998. 'Women's Desires and Burden: Family Planning in Northeast Thailand', *Asian Studies Review* 22(2): 137–55.
———. 1999. 'Birth and the Postpartum in Northeast Thailand: Contesting Modernity and Tradition', *Medical Anthropology: Cross-Cultural Studies in Health and Illness* 18(3): 215–42.
———. 2000. *Intimate Knowledge: Women and Their Health in Northeast Thailand.* Sydney: Allen and Unwin.
———. 2002a. 'Water Serpents and Staying by the Fire: Markers of Maturity in a Northeast Thai Village', in L. Manderson and P. Liamputtong Rice (eds.), *Coming of Age: Adolescence in South-East Asia.* London: NIAS/Curzon, 17–41.
——— (ed.). 2002b. *Women's Health in Mainland Southeast Asia.* Binghamton, NY: Haworth Medical Press.
———. 2004. *Abortion, Sin and the State in Thailand.* London: Routledge Curzon.
———. 2008. 'Pleasure and Pain: Medical Travel in Asia', *Global Public Health: An International Journal for Research, Policy and Practice* 33(3): 271–90.
———. 2009. 'Global Technologies and Transnational Reproduction in Thailand', *Asian Studies Review* 33(3): 319–32.

———. 2010. 'Challenges of Medical Travel to Global Regulation: A Case Study of Reproductive Travel in Asia', *Global Social Policy* 10(3): 287–91.

———. 2011. 'Cross-Border Assisted Reproductive Care in Asia: Implications for Access, Equity and Regulations', *Reproductive Health Matters* 19(37): 107–16.

———. 2012. 'Cross-Border Assisted Reproductive Care: Global Quests for a Child', in J. R. Hodges, L. Turner and A. M. Kimball (eds.), *Risks and Challenges in Medical Tourism: Understanding the Global Market for Health Services.* Santa Barbara, CA: Praeger, 167–86.

Wilson, A. 2008. 'The Sacred Geography of Bangkok's Markets', *International Journal of Urban and Regional Research* 32(3): 631–42.

Zegers-Hochschild, F., J. E. Schwarze and V. Alam. 2008. 'Infertility', in K. Heggenhougen and S. Quah (eds.), *International Encyclopedia of Public Health.* Waltham, MA: Academic Press, 576–87.

INDEX